LATIN AMERICAN STUDIES
SOCIAL SCIENCES AND LAW

Edited by
David Mares
University of California, San Diego

A ROUTLEDGE SERIES

LATIN AMERICAN STUDIES

DAVID MARES, *General Editor*

AN INDUSTRIAL GEOGRAPHY
OF COCAINE

Christian M. Allen

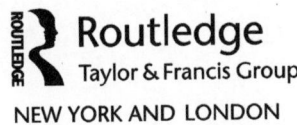

Routledge
Taylor & Francis Group

NEW YORK AND LONDON

Published in 2005 by
Routledge
605 Third Avenue,
New York, NY 10017

Published in Great Britain by
Routledge
2 Park Square
Milton Park, Abingdon
Oxon OX14 4RN

Routledge is an imprint of the Taylor & Francis Group, an informa business

Library of Congress Cataloging-in-Publication Data

Allen, Christian Michael.
  An industrial geography of cocaine / Christian Michael Allen.
    p. cm. -- (Latin American studies: social sciences and law)
  Includes bibliographical references and index.
  ISBN 0-415-94940-8 (hardback : alk. paper)
  1. Cocaine industry--Latin America. 2. Cocaine
industry--Location--Latin America. I. Title. II. Series : Latin
American studies (Routledge (Firm)). Social sciences and law.

  HV5840.L3A63 2005
  363.45'098--dc22
                                                        2005018133

ISBN13: 978-0-415-94940-8 (hbk)
ISBN13: 978-0-415-80490-5 (pbk)

Contents

List of Figures

List of Photos

List of Tables

Acknowledgments

No project of this scope could be completed without the support, encouragement, information, and advice provided by a number of individuals and institutions. I must first thank my colleagues in geography at the University of Cincinnati, especially Robert South, Howard Stafford, Nicholas Dunning and Robert Frohn. Thomas Moore of the Department of Political Science at Cincinnati also played an important guiding role for this study. Your comments, questions, advice, and friendship are all appreciated.

I wish to express my gratitude to the following individuals for their generosity in time, knowledge, and materials: John Eck of the Division of Criminal Justice at Cincinnati; Santos Ramirez and Alfonso Moreno of the U.S. Border Patrol; Dewey Owens and Fred Ball of the Office of National Drug Control Policy; Mark Langenderfer of the U.S. Customs Service; Marc Flicker of the Defense Intelligence Agency; John Tomasovich of the National Imagery and Mapping Agency; Carlos Sarabia Blanco, Cesar Castellon, and Oscar Antezana of USAID; Roberto Laserna of the Centro de Estudios de la Realidad Economica y Social in Cochabamba, Bolivia; the RAND Corporation; and Tony Newman and Matt Briggs of the Lindesmith Center. My relationships with you have considerably enriched the model of the cocaine trade presented here.

Finally, I wish to thank my family and friends for their interest, encouragement, and support - this work is dedicated to you all. I am particularly obliged to my parents for promoting from an early age my interest in the world beyond our doorstep. I am equally grateful to Stephanie for serving as my primary sounding board throughout this project and for her unique understanding of my personal commitment to it. For Elizabeth, Natalie, and Noah, my hope is that by the time you are old enough to read this, we'll have implemented a more constructive and compassionate drug policy regime.

Chapter One

Through the Lens of Economic Geography: Cocaine in Space and Place

The production and marketing of cocaine has a great deal in common with the sales of legal products. The transferability of skills and technology from legitimate business enterprises to drug trafficking has spurred its development into a modern trans-national industry. Latin American trafficking organizations hold significant competitive advantages in the industry, owing to their effective use of local factor endowments. Their success stands in stark contrast to the limited success that the region's licit firms have had in international markets.

Trafficking organizations have developed impressive industrial, financial, transportation, intelligence, and communications networks on an international scale. This infrastructure reflects the exceptional degree of organization and expertise required to manufacture and distribute an illicit good valued in the tens of billions of dollars a year. The industry's success in generating foreign exchange earnings means that the actors comprising it can wield significant influence over political and economic institutions at all levels throughout Latin America (Lee, 1999: 6).

The recent and widespread adoption of market-oriented economic reforms throughout the region has re-drawn its economic, political, and social landscape (Brohman, 1996; Otero, 1996; Kay 1993). Drug trafficking organizations (DTOs) have demonstrated unusual success in their response to these new and challenging conditions. Their export strategies are inspired by the development policies recommended by international lending organizations like the World Bank (Castells, 1998: 173). Indeed, Andreas (1999a: 125) has described Mexican drug trafficking organizations as "the quintessential expression of the kind of private sector entrepreneurialism celebrated and encouraged by neoliberal economic orthodoxy." Moreover, such policies encourage expanded flows of international trade and capital, which, in turn, offer DTOs many opportunities to exploit licit channels to move product and profits across borders. Such opportunities reflect a fundamental tension between the two broad policy regimes that most influence the cocaine trade. Exploring the nexus of economic liberalization and drug prohibition is a secondary objective of this research.

The primary objective is to model the cocaine industry and its firms. The cocaine trade has attracted a great deal of popular attention, yet remains poorly understood. A huge volume of relevant information exists, (especially from state sources) but it is poorly organized and too often isolated from meaningful context. This research generates a conceptual model of cocaine production and distribution, one that reflects Chorley and Haggett's (1967: 21) catholic view of models–that they need not be a theory, law, or equation, but rather a structured idea or synthesis of data. It seeks to place the cocaine trade within a meaningful context, by helping the reader understand the economic, social, and political landscape within which DTOs act. This is accomplished by disintegrating the cocaine industry into its functional stages (from the cultivation of coca leaf at its source to marketing operations in the United States) and assessing each individually. In the concluding chapter, the component stages are re-integrated and the cocaine business is considered as a whole.

Drug trafficking organizations operate in and across space much like licit firms. While criminal enterprises face a more complex and uncertain landscape, their potential responses to the challenges and opportunities presented by space and place are fundamentally no different than those of licit firms. Models developed to explain firm behavior in licit industries are no less applicable when applied to an illegal economic activity. Models borrowed from economic geography facilitate the development of normative structures used to evaluate cocaine industry processes. They play an important guiding role in the categorization and classification system used to organize the data collected for this research. Finally, they help to fill gaps in knowledge about the cocaine trade that result from poor or insufficient data.

Glasmeier (2000) and Dicken (1998) produce valuable explanations of industrial development across space and time, demonstrating the descriptive and analytical value of many of the organizing principles applied in this research to the cocaine industry. Rengert (1996) conclusively demonstrated the utility of geographic models for enhancing understanding of the drug trade. A narrow focus on downstream marketing stages limits the potential contribution of his approach, however. Extending the use of location theory and modeling to the entire production and distribution chain provides valuable insight regarding the strategic decision-making process of business enterprises (Hanink, 1997; Hayter, 1997; Jones and Simmons, 1990).

The notion of competitive advantage details the links between firm and industry-specific determinants of success and the location-specific characteristics from which they are derived (Porter, 1990). It helps explain the complex interplay between firm and place, and is therefore an invaluable (yet under-appreciated) tool for modeling the spatial organization of industrial systems (Grant, 1994). It is used in this research to evaluate how different home environments influence the development of drug trafficking organizations. DTOs commonly pursue functional specialization in a relatively small subset of industry activities, often focusing on just one. The scope and functional orientation of any DTO reflect relevant local conditions.

Additional insight is provided through corporate geography, which explains location decisions by the factors that influence strategy formulation. It is a normative approach incorporating a variety of factors that influence firm behavior (Laulajainen, 1995). Factors internal to the firm include its motivations, expertise and existing spatial structure. State policy, market conditions, and the strategies of rival and supplier firms are all significant external influences. Thus, the formulation of successful firm strategies must incorporate the firm's own 'inertia,' the anticipated behavior of other organizations, and the general economic climate. The strategies a firm decides to pursue both reflect and influence its spatial organization (Dicken and Lloyd, 1990).

It is important to remember that all the models used in this research are subjective approximations of reality that do not include all observations. Their value lies in obscuring incidental detail while presenting significant features or relationships in a generalized form (Chorley and Haggett, 1967: 220). Geographic models are employed here as guiding principles that illuminate the spatial form and behavior of drug trafficking organizations. Their application to a unique, non-traditional industry provides original and valuable insight into the operations of a poorly understood business. Models are not used here to generate formal, equation-based, quantitative descriptions of industry processes. The available data is neither sufficiently comprehensive nor reliable enough to warrant such an approach.

DATA

The model developed in this research is primarily of a qualitative nature, as quantitative model development is hampered by an almost total lack of relevant firm-scale data. Considering the illicit and secretive nature of the industry, such information is understandably difficult to collect (Laserna, 1995b: 25). The figures used to describe the production, transportation, marketing, and consumption of drugs are little more than 'guesstimates,' subject to critical interpretation (Economist, 2001d: 3). A joint State Department-USAID report on the cocaine trade in Bolivia reflects this troublesome fact:

> A number of guesses and estimates have been used in the absence of precise information. Resulting values are very approximate and should be interpreted accordingly (see Holden-Rhodes, 1997: 149).

Further obstacles to quantitative modeling are inconsistencies over space and time in the methods used to collect and present drug-related data. Different countries and their numerous law enforcement and intelligence institutions pursue unique goals and maintain individual standards, making it difficult to reconcile their figures into a comprehensive picture. Worse yet, these standards are subject to change (commonly without explanation) even over short time periods. Discrepancies over space and through time suggest that estimates are used as much to support political objectives, demonstrate the efficacy of law enforcement efforts, or justify funding levels as much as they are to provide an accurate reflection of industry conditions (see Laserna, 1997: 203–212). Even the Office of National Drug Control Policy notes: "Drug smuggling is . . . not easily subject to controlled research conditions (ONDCP, 2000: 3).

Using less charitable terms, Reuter (1996: 63–64) describes:

> an essentially madcap series of federal figures on international production and prices that make a mockery of the whole enterprise. These estimates and their components are so inconsistent and erratic that they demonstrate what might reasonably be called a "reckless disregard" for the truth. . . . the numbers are in fact just decorations on the policy process, rhetorical conveniences for official statements without any serious consequences.

Despite these limitations, reports produced by the anti-narcotics intelligence units of federal agencies such as the Departments of State, Justice, and Commerce remain an important source of data used in this research. While it is necessary to recognize the limitations of such sources, it is a mistake to dismiss them entirely. Over-simplified estimates of coca cultivation, cocaine production, interdiction rates, or consumption deserve skepticism, yet the abundant qualitative observations contained in these sources are essential to the description and model-building objectives of this research.

Counter-narcotics expert Holden-Rhodes (1997:152) argues in favor of a qualitative approach for research into drug trafficking, as a balance against the 'body count' mentality prevalent in existing anti-drug intelligence. This attitude reflects an obsession with flawed quantitative measures of the cocaine trade like the amount of land cultivated in coca, its yield, conversion rates for the refining process, or the volume shipped to the United States. While some criticize qualitative research as 'story-telling,' "a qualitative approach is intellectually rigorous and . . . concerned with the quality of the knowledge it produces (Schoenberger, 1992: 216)." Rigor in qualitative research comes from a process of 'triangulation' involving the use multiple sources, methods, and theories (Bradshaw and Stratford, 2000: 47).

The bibliography contains a complete list of official sources used, but a sampling of the most important is provided here. These incorporate qualitative treatments of drug production and trafficking activity, as well as raw quantitative data and related models of cocaine production, distribution, or consumption.

- National Drug Intelligence Center, 2001. *National Drug Threat Assessment*
- ONDCP, 2000. *Estimation of Cocaine Availability*
- Federal Drug Information Center, 2000. *International Crime Threat Assessment*
- Dept. of State, 1995–2000. *International Narcotics Control Strategy Report*
- Drug Enforcement Agency, 1999. *Briefing Book*
- ONDCP, 1997. *What America's Users Spend on Illegal Drugs*
- USAID, 1997. *Bolivia's Coca-Cocaine Sub-Economy: A Computer Model*
- National Narcotics Intelligence Consumers Committee, 1996. *The Supply of Illicit Drugs to the U.S.*

Additional information was generated through a series of open-ended interviews with officials from the Office of National Drug Control Policy, Drug Enforcement Agency, Border Patrol, Customs Service, Defense Intelligence Agency, National Imagery and Mapping Agency, and U.S. Aid for International Development. While these contacts rarely produced formal quantitative databases, the discussions provided a rich context in which to place and better understand the raw information acquired from the open sources detailed above. Unstructured interviews explore lines of inquiry in a flexible manner and are an important source of information for intensive research (Hayter, 1997: 11). Clark (1998: 73) argues that this 'close dialogue' method is a useful means of promoting conceptual innovation in economic geography. In most cases, the interviewees did not extend permission to the author to formally cite these discussions.

Another major source of data used in this research is the existing body of academic books and articles offering description, models, or analysis of the drug trade and associated themes. Such works contribute immeasurably to the scope, depth, and relevance of the contextual landscape developed in this project. A few of the most important sources of this type include:

- Andreas, 2000. *Border Games: Policing the U.S.- Mexico Divide*
- Friman and Andreas, 1999. *The Illicit Global Economy and State Power*
- Jacobs, 1999. *Dealing Crack: The Social World of Streetcorner Selling*
- Farer (ed.), 1999. *Transnational Crime in the Americas*
- Holden-Rhodes, 1997. *Sharing the Secrets: Open Source Intelligence and the War on Drugs*
- Clawson and Lee, 1996. *The Andean Cocaine Industry*
- Rengert, 1996. *The Geography of Illegal Drugs*
- Riley, 1996. *Snow Job? The War against International Cocaine Trafficking*
- Thoumi, 1995. *Political Economy & Illegal Drugs in Colombia*
- Dombrey-Moore (et.al.), 1994. *A System Description of the Cocaine Trade*
- Painter, 1994. *Bolivia and Coca: A Study in Dependency*
- Kennedy (et. al.), 1993. *A Simple Economic Model of Cocaine Production*

The final source of data for this project is hundreds of magazine and newspaper articles from international news services. The quantity and quality of coverage by *The Economist* on drug-related issues in Latin America is particularly noteworthy. News articles add valuable 'local' detail to the author's understanding of the cocaine trade. The majority of the material collected in support of this research can be considered 'open source.' The lack of access to classified materials does not in any way devalue the conclusions reached here. Products generated from open source intelligence are commonly valued for their scope, depth, and for the accuracy of their findings and forecasts (Holden-Rhodes, 1997: 100).

ANALYSIS IN ECONOMIC GEOGRAPHY

Source material for this project totals tens of thousands of pages. This volume of information must be critically evaluated and refined in order to produce meaningful conclusions about the cocaine trade. This filtering process is guided by a series of organizing principles that determine how information is selected, analyzed, and presented. The explicit focus of this research is the spatial organization of the cocaine industry and its component firms, therefore its organizing principles reflect the theoretical models commonly used to explain the form and behavior of economic activities in space.

> from its beginnings the central tasks of industrial geography have been, and remain, to explain the location of industrial activity, changes in the location of industrial activity, and the implications of changing patterns of industrial location for national, regional, and local economic development (Hayter, 1997: xiii).

No single model can account for the dynamism and variability found in economic systems. Accordingly, this research uses a variety of conceptual tools and research methods: neoclassical location theory, behavioral approaches to location decision-making, corporate geography, central place theory, spatial diffusion, and the notion of competitive advantage each offer explanatory value in the context of the cocaine trade. This approach generates a diverse set of theoretical constructs that organizes and integrates the body of qualitative and quantitative data collected in support of this research. Reliance on contributions from different theoretical perspectives reflects the fact that business organizations are "socially complex and densely spatial objects of analysis" that are messier than our theories of them (Del Casino, et.al., 2000: 535).

The approach used here reflects a recent trend towards theoretical pluralism in economic geography (Wai-chung 2000: 301). What has emerged to prominence is a qualitative and speculative mode of analysis that seeks to portray the spatial scope and diversity of economic systems (Clark, 1998: 74). It recognizes that the development of economic systems in time and space does not result simply from 'geographic' processes like the friction of distance, but also from wider economic, political, and cultural contexts (Barnes, 2001: 558; Wai-chung, 2000: 308; Wai-chung, 1994: 475; Dicken and Lloyd, 1990: 9). A postmodern approach maintains a creative tension between diverse intellectual traditions to produce better interpretations (Forbes, 2000; 139; Dear, 1988: 271). While theory in the economic geography may lack a single source, form, or final empirical means of proof, it can nonetheless reveal the world (specifically its economic landscape) in persuasive and compelling ways (Barnes, 2001).

Schoenberger (1992) and Dear (1988: 268) aver that research is really about interpretation rather than revealed facts or undebatable truths. Barnes (2001) takes a similar view, lauding the recent growth of what he calls 'hermeneutic' theorizing in geography, which emphasizes open-ended, interpretive accounts. As Barnes (1988: 349) argued, "there is no Industrial Geography, only industrial geographies." The title of this project, *An Industrial Geography of Cocaine,* reflects such concerns. It claims neither perfect information nor comprehensiveness and recognizes that alternative approaches and explanations exist. The text contains assertions that are not documented with unassailable evidence. Some are based on information provided by interview sources who did not wish to be formally cited. For the most part, however, these are personal interpretations based on analysis of gathered observations or empirical fieldwork. They reflect the clandestine nature of the cocaine industry and the resulting paucity of irrefutable evidence. More importantly, they demonstrate the informal, intuitive, and often overlooked nature of much geographical analysis (Goodchild, 1992: 142). As Sauer (1963: 403) noted:

> Beyond all that can be communicated by instruction and mastered by techniques lies a realm of individual perception and interpretation, the art of geography.

The limited spatial scope of this work is a further argument against considering it *The* definitive geography of cocaine. No attempt is made here to describe or analyze the development of Europe's growing cocaine market, itself a meaningful industrial geography. Rather, its contribution is to provide an original view of the pan-American core of the cocaine business through the penetrating lens of economic geography.

A critical first step in this research process is the development of comprehensive descriptions of the phenomena under study. Lewis (1985: 469) argues that good science begins with a solid accumulation of facts, carefully described. Sayer (1982: 78) contends that much research is actually not directly concerned with explanation. Rather, its purpose is to gather and communicate information about a particular situation. Certainly, description plays an important integrating and summarizing role; one that

> strip(s) away unnecessary detail and delineate(s) more clearly the central characteristics of the data. Moreover, it is in pulling together and relating these central characteristics through a reasoned account that description acquires its unity and force (Dey, 1993: 39)

Of course, good science goes beyond description. The model developed here incorporates the analytical rigor of a wide body of theory from economic geography and related disciplines. It examines drug trafficking organizations as multinational business enterprises, focusing on their organization and behavior in space. Yet multinationals do not exploit space per se, rather the varied material and social environments in different times and places (Sayer, 1985:53). The strategic decisions made by DTOs therefore reflect the challenges and opportunities presented by a dynamic economic, social, and political landscape.

This research relies in large part upon 'relational' explanation, which relates a phenomenon in need of explanation to other events of which we already have an understanding, either through familiarity or analysis (Harvey, 1969: 14; Chorley and Haggett, 1967: 24). In this type of explanation, the critical task is to provide a network of connections between relevant events and processes associated with both the 'familiar' and the 'unfamiliar' phenomena. In this research, these are the behavior of licit economic actors and the behavior of DTOs, respectively.

> Geographers approach the study of manufacturing from a viewpoint that emphasizes either firms or places. When firms are of primary significance, interest focuses on the locational choices that firms make. When areas are emphasized, attention centers on the nature of industries in a city, a region, or a country (Stutz and de Souza, 1988: 344).

This project values both perspectives. It examines the behavior of DTOs in space: the spatial organization of a firm's component parts, as well as the management of multinational business operations. It places equal emphasis on the role of place in the development of the cocaine trade. Particular countries, regions, and cities have long been associated with industry success; the location conditions that attract or sustain specific drug related activities are the explicit focus here. Choosing one or the other viewpoint unnecessarily limits the scope and potential contribution of the research. Rather, industrial geography should develop an understanding of the complex dynamic *between* firm and place.

To that end, this research incorporates a strong idiographic element, embedded within case studies of Bolivia, Colombia, and Mexico in Chapters 3, 4, and 5. Each is conceptually organized around a set of research questions that address complex and situated thematic issues. They are an invaluable tool for illuminating specific, local manifestations of the broader theoretical and policy issues addressed throughout this research. Clark (1998: 75) argues that case studies are valuable research tools in economic geography, for they facilitate an appreciation for the diversity of economic systems. All cases have unique, important, and interesting features which deserve elaboration. Warren (1970: viii) notes,

> analysis in economic geography requires a resolution to probe as far as possible into the reasons for location decisions, . . . and to look into the contingencies of industry and company development.

Yet the examination of the particular competes with the need for generalization, with too much focus on the atypical diminishing the process of theory building. By maintaining an appropriate level of generalization, case studies are useful both for refining theory and suggesting complexities for further investigation (Stake, 2000: 448).

The case studies in this research focus on the location-specific characteristics of 'local' environments and their influence on the development of the cocaine business there. The context in which a phenomenon occurs is important not only because it situates the action, but also in the way it aids in understanding the broader social and historical significance (Dey, 1993: 32).

The first case study focuses on the cultivation of coca and the manufacturing of cocaine in Bolivia. It identifies important location factors for coca cultivation and processing facilities, details the industry's competitive structure and spatial organization, and examines implications for economic development. The second illuminates the historically dominant position of Colombian firms in the cocaine trade. It evaluates the unique package of location-specific social, political, and economic characteristics that contribute to a favorable business climate for DTOs. The final case study examines the critical role of Mexican traffickers in the trans-shipment of cocaine from producer nations to the United States. It focuses on how a favorable location encourages the development of internationally competitive firms at the smuggling and wholesale distribution stages of the production chain. The most important feature of this environment is the U.S.-Mexico border, which receives detailed treatment.

QUALITATIVE DATA ANALYSIS

Qualitative data analysis encompasses a variety of approaches related to the specific goals and disciplinary perspectives of the researcher. It is an interpretative, open-ended and creative process that is often difficult to describe explicitly (Barnes, 2001: 551; Dey, 1993: 5; Strauss, 1987: 4). It is a process undertaken not through prescription, but as an art (Kitchin and Tate, 2000: 229). The common task of the varied approaches to qualitative data analysis are filtering and categorizing an unstructured mass of information to make it more suggestive and easier to interpret. By organizing the data into a coherent argument, it makes the volume of information accessible to readers who did not participate in collection and analysis (Clark, 1998: 79).

Qualitative methods are often called 'intensive' research, for they involve in-depth analysis of how processes operate in the context of specific cases (Bradshaw and Stratford, 2000: 40). They seek to produce 'thick' description—a comprehensive account of an event or action, including information regarding the situational context, the intentions of the actors, and a description of the process within which the situation is embedded (Berg and Mansvelt, 2000: 177; Kitchin and Tate, 2000: 233). The goal is to introduce the rich texture of local circumstances that have been ignored by theorists more concerned with simplicity than diversity in economic systems (Clark, 1998: 82). Intensive research documents

> distinctive and unusually important processes which cannot be effectively subjected to extensive research and can illuminate arguments and debates over alternatives that would otherwise remain uncovered (Hayter, 1997: 11).

The rich and complex nature of qualitative data forces the researcher to decide what data are relevant and how to interpret them. One must identify themes and meaning while selecting some pieces of information as more pertinent than others. The first step towards interpretation is classification, a creative process that removes data from its original context, providing new ways to think about it (Kinchin and Tate, 2000: 239). Dey (1993: 94) notes that we

> create conceptual tools to classify and compare the important or essential features of the phenomena we are studying. This involves a process of abstracting from the immense detail and complexity of our data those features which are most salient for our purpose.

Classification organizes and facilitates the analysis of data, while preventing the researcher from becoming overwhelmed by the sheer volume of data or immersed in anecdotes. This process depends not only on inferences from the data, but also the imagination, intuition, and previous knowledge of the researcher (Dey, 1993: 100).

Classification is the most basic form of analysis, grouping events and observations by identifying commonalities and divergences (Goodchild, 1992: 152). Data within groups is examined for similarities and differences, and further differentiated if necessary. Categories are developed using a set of criteria that distinguish some observations from others. Such schemes must reflect both a relevant conceptual context as well as an empirical reality (Kinchin and Tate, 2000: 245). This process generates a conceptual framework that reflects the original research questions, as well as the substantive, policy, and theoretical issues they imply. Classification

> provides a means of building up a general picture of the observed world, bridging local observation with broader interests and concerns, and thereby *making* a world rather than simply accepting as given a *ready-made* world composed by theorists (Clark, 1998: 79).

Qualitative analysis is an iterative process, continually returning to and revising earlier analysis as the evidence becomes more clearly organized and understood. As categories are refined into a conceptual framework, gaps in the data are identified. These holes are filled through the collection of precise information that illuminates the emerging theory. Redundant data gathering minimizes the likelihood of misinterpreting data patterns. Observations are interpreted against one theme or perspective, then against others, in an attempt to revise and refine meanings and relationships (Stake, 2000: 443–5).

> The process of qualitative analysis is much like being a detective. You have the accounts from a number of sources which you then need to piece together and try to determine what is going on (Kinchin and Tate, 2000: 251).

After the initial classification, the assumptions underlying the conceptual framework are elaborated. Comparisons are made within and between groups and sub-groups in an attempt to identify patterns in the data. Charmaz (2000: 517) notes, "raw data from different sources provide the grist for making precise comparisons, fleshing out ideas, analyzing properties of categories, and seeing patterns." The goal is to understand the nature of relationships between data—how they are associated (separate events occurring together) and how they interact (engagement between two events) (Kinchin and Tate, 2000: 247). Connections between categories and their relation to larger processes are defined, a process linking analytical interpretation with empirical reality.

> It is precisely a qualitative discrimination between different types of relations and an identification of the connections between specific mechanisms and their particular conditions that is needed for explanation (Sayer, 1982: 76).

Qualitative analysis can produce a variety of interpretations and will sometimes fail to address ambiguities in the explanations of the processes under analysis. Such efforts are nonetheless worthwhile, as observation and formalized description contribute greatly to our understanding of spatial processes (Goodchild, 1992).

The first task of this research is to develop the conceptual framework for analyzing cocaine trafficking organizations as multi-national corporations. The following chapter does so by evaluating the impact of market-based economic reforms on the industry, the adoption of international business strategies by its 'firms,' relevant location conditions and the determinants of competitive advantage, and the price structure, sources of value added, and role of innovation in the cocaine business. The next four chapters provide examples of how such considerations manifest themselves in the various functional stages and places that comprise the cocaine trade. Chapter seven addresses the myriad policy implications that arise from the study of an illicit industry. Considering the important role state policy plays in the cocaine trade, to ignore these issues would be a critical omission. The concluding chapter reassembles the production and distribution chain to promote explanations of the spatial patterns and location decision-making in the industry as a whole. It also evaluates the utility of the methodological approaches used in the research and provides and industry forecast for the near future.

Chapter Two
Globalization and the Competitive Strategies of Criminal Enterprises

Over the past three decades, the accelerated development of a deep and complex form of internationalization has become the primary influence on economics throughout the globe. This *globalization* is an uneven transition process from an international economy comprised of discrete national units to a global economy of integrated national economies. The production and distribution of goods and services are increasingly organized across national boundaries, and industries of all types are oriented towards global markets. Three broad trends underlie this shift: an international political economy committed to reducing the role of the state in economic affairs; a time-space convergence brought about by improvements in transportation technology and infrastructure, and an increased capacity for the collection and processing of information, made possible by advances in telecommunications and computing.

Market-oriented economic reforms seek to reduce state intervention in markets, which are seen as causing price distortions, macroeconomic imbalances, and misallocation of resources. Proponents argue that the state is a hindrance to development and that nations are better off abandoning state-led, inward-oriented development programs (Brohman, 1996: 108). Policies promoting economic liberalization include:

- Removing controls on capital movements and deregulating banking.
- Privatizing state-owned enterprises and eliminating government subsidies.
- Facilitating cross-border trade by removing tariff and non-tariff barriers.
- Export-led development strategies, with economic specialization based on competitive advantage.

The widespread adoption of such policies (in conjunction with the technological advances mentioned earlier) has generated considerable growth in social, political, and economic interactions of all types between places. Such exchanges are commonly conceptualized in terms of increased flows of people, information, commodities, and capital across borders. Yet globalization is also qualitatively different from earlier forms of international exchange. More important than increased 'flows' is the functional integration of economic activities and 'national' economies across borders (Dicken, 1998). This cross-border restructuring stimulates the development of strategic alliances by business enterprises (Portnoy, 2000:157).

The increasing volume of cross-border exchange (often in conjunction with streamlined regulatory procedures) provides many opportunities to hide contraband in licit flows. In this manner, globalization has facilitated the international movement of illicit commodities and profits (McCaffery, 1999: 5). The implementation of NAFTA, for example, has eased the movement of large drug shipments into the U.S. and solidified the strong position of Mexican DTOs in the industry (Andreas, 1999a). The rise of major Colombian DTOs took place amidst Colombia's own economic liberalization efforts, which encouraged cross-border flows of trade and investment. These flows provide the cocaine business with numerous opportunities to conceal their operations and launder money behind the cover of legitimate businesses (Thoumi, 1999: 127). By facilitating cross-border economic activities, regional free-market reforms have played a similarly important role in the development of trafficking alliances throughout the Caribbean (Maingot, 1999).

Criminal organizations have expanded the spatial scope of their activities, linking actors across international borders through functional networks. For this reason, crime is a complex trans-sovereign problem that individual states cannot alone control. The regulatory mechanisms of global markets are highly fragmented, creating numerous opportunities for criminal actors to exploit a variety of 'criminogenic' asymmetries (Passas, 2001:23). These asymmetries stimulate demand for illicit commodities, create incentives to engage in illegal markets, and reduce the capacity of the state to respond to such activities. State institutions are increasingly challenged by a tension between promoting free market capitalism while simultaneously restricting the flow of drugs, arms, prostitutes, 'conflict' diamonds, or other undesirable commodities.

Yet to suggest that globalization has diminished state sovereignty is too simple. While weak states have certainly experienced a considerable decline in sovereignty, stronger states have not. Indeed, strong states play active roles in constructing globalization through their influence on the discourse of transnational institutions (Herod, et. al, 1998: 14). The more accurate conclusion is that the role of the state in 'core' countries has changed, but not necessarily diminished. States remain the most important actors in the regulation of markets, the reconstruction of borders, and the development and enforcement of prohibition regimes. It is through these decisions that states contribute to defining the 'illicit spaces' of economies (Farer; 1999: 251).

COMPETITIVE ADVANTAGE

Globalization processes are complex, contested, and difficult to identify and measure. They are simultaneously social, political, and economic, dependent on local contingencies, and thus unevenly developed over space and time (Hay and Marsh, 2000: 3). Specific local characteristics interact with global processes to generate distinct outcomes. All manner of organizations and enterprises, including criminal ones, are rooted in some particular 'local' set of conditions and institutions that shape their opportunities, goals, and means (Castells, 2000: 188). Their study should take into account these physical, social and historical dimensions of their development in space and time. Yeung (1994: 475) argues that

> By recognizing the cultural and social *embeddedness* of the formation of network relations and economic transactions, we can arrive at a better understanding of the nature of production systems prevailing in different societies and localities.

Multinational enterprises reflect their home country environments, where they remain strongly embedded (Dicken, 1998: 178), an observation that Castells (1998: 197) makes regarding DTOs as well. Prominent traffickers emerged in favorable national 'home bases' where they have been able to create competitive advantages in trafficking and related activities. Here, the organization's essential and proprietary skills reside and strategy and product development take place.

Porter's (1990) model of competitive advantage offers an illustrative conceptual framework for considering the pursuit of embedded advantages by cocaine trafficking organizations. He identifies four 'determinants' of competitive advantage that each vary unevenly across space, and therefore have profound implications for the development of economic activities in any particular place. Different industries are structured through unique sets of underlying economic and technical characteristics, and therefore have different requirements for success (Porter, 1990: 36). Some nations provide better environments for competing in some industries (or industry sectors) than others. Porter's determinants include factor conditions; demand conditions, related and supporting industries; and the nature of firm strategy, structure and rivalry. Sustainable competitive advantage typically results from overlapping strengths in multiple determinants.

Yet firms do not derive their advantages merely from operating in a favorable environment. They must *create* firm-scale competitive advantages by developing business strategies that capitalize on these favorable characteristics of their 'home bases' (Porter, 1990). Examples of created advantage include Japanese automobile manufacturers, who pioneered lean production methods in the 1970s (Dicken, 1998: 325–342), and watch producers based in Hong-Kong, who exploited the introduction of quartz technology to claim dominance in low-end market sectors (Glasmeier, 2000: 216–231). This research examines created competitive advantage in the cocaine trade, by identifying the local influence of spatially differentiated 'determinants.' Competitive advantage at the various stages of cocaine's production and distribution chain relies on different combinations of determinants. Therefore, the functional orientation the cocaine industry in any particular place reflects local conditions. Case studies of Bolivia, Colombia, and Mexico in subsequent chapters each offer valuable insight regarding how local environments shape the competitive advantages of 'home' DTOs.

The first determinant, factor conditions, includes a variety of physical, human, knowledge, and capital resources. In the cocaine trade, valuable physical resources include large stretches of remote territory with minimal state presence, environmental conditions favoring coca cultivation, proximity to important markets, or access to natural smuggling channels. Relevant human resources include deep pools of peasant and/or relevant professional labor. Knowledge resources are especially important for creating advantage in marketing functions and are generated through a network of contacts, informants, and specialists. These might include knowledge of processing innovations, market conditions, or counter-intelligence in response to law enforcement efforts. Strong capital resources allow DTOs to develop human and physical infrastructure for executing processing, distribution, and intelligence functions. Trafficking organizations in Colombia and Mexico, for example, benefited from their more highly developed national economies and banking systems. In these places, sufficient capital is available for illicit ventures and the repatriation and laundering of proceeds is easier and less costly.

Firms gain competitive advantage through their 'local' access to low cost or high quality resources relative to competitors in their industry. Yet these resources must also be recognized and efficiently exploited by local enterprises. Such profitable exploitation of favorable factor endowments by drug trafficking organizations occurs in 'home' business climates where pressure to innovate, improve, and expand are greatest. The process of identifying and implementing innovative business strategies is manifest in "product changes, process changes, new approaches to marketing, new forms of distribution, and new conceptions of scope (Porter, 1990: 45)."

Stimuli for such innovations include technological developments, changes in market size or structure, shifts in the availability or cost of inputs, the actions of competitors, and government regulation. The latter are particularly relevant to the cocaine trade, and clearly reflect Porter's (1990: 83) contention that "pressure instead of abundance or a comfortable environment underpins true competitive advantage." Law enforcement efforts targeting DTOs stimulate firm innovation and adaptation, just as product standards, trade barriers or other regulatory regimes do in licit industries.

The importance of competition as a foundation for competitive advantage is evident in the savage domestic rivalries that commonly exist among DTOs. Vigorous domestic rivalries are a key to the development and sustainability of competitive advantage at the international scale because they create pressure to innovate. Firms must develop new technologies or processes, exploit economies of scale, fine-tune their distribution channels, or take advantage of favorable home nation characteristics better than their competitors. Porter (1990: 119) notes,

> it is rare that a company can meet tough foreign rivals when it has faced no significant competition at home . . . Rivalry among domestic firms often goes beyond the purely economic and can become emotional and even personal. Active feuds between domestic rivals are common, and often associated with an internationally successful national industry.

Such feuds are a common feature of the cocaine trade, particularly in Colombia and Mexico, where dozens of family-based major and minor DTOs operate in a tangled web of alliances and vicious rivalries (Bowden, 2001; Gray, 1998; Holden-Rhodes, 1997 Oppenheimer, 1996; Clawson and Lee, 1996; Thoumi, 1995).

The presence and sophistication of related and supporting industries is another important determinant of competitive advantage. All firms exist in a system of 'value chains' linking upstream and downstream industries (Porter, 1990: 42). Firms create competitive advantage when they manage these external links in a way that 'internalizes' other firms' advantages. If a value system is composed of many competitive firms, these advantages are more easily realized. A number of related industrial sectors influence the development of competitive advantage in the cocaine trade. These include: coca cultivation, producers and distributors of precursor chemicals; cocaine refiners; transportation brokers; intelligence and security specialists; and financial services.

The third determinant includes a set of social, political, and economic characteristics that govern the organization and management of firms, social norms of individual and group behaviors, and professional standards. The influence of such characteristics on the development of the pan-American cocaine trade is best illustrated by the Colombian firms that have dominated the industry since the 1970s cocaine boom, in part because of their extraordinary capacity for ruthlessness and violence (see Thoumi, 1995). In illicit markets, regulation and the settlement of disputes are often managed through the targeted application of violence. Colombian DTOs are infamous for their routine and effective use of this "management tool." Such violence also acts as a significant barrier to potential market entrants. New participants commonly lack sufficient resources, risk tolerance, or the capacity to use violence as a tool in the pursuit of business goals. Because of these deficiencies, established competitors often eliminate newcomers before they can position themselves (Castells, 1998: 193). Business related violence is often intra-national; Colombian DTOs, for instance, target other Colombian groups as they struggle to control access to raw materials or smuggling channels (Drexler, 1997: 161). Other good examples include the turf battles fought by Mexican DTOs over lucrative cross-border smuggling routes (Padgett and Shannon, 2001, Smith, 1999; Oppenheimer, 1996).

While domestic demand for cocaine is relatively small in producer and distributor nations, demand conditions remain an important determinant. The greatest demand is in the United States and nations with 'preferential' access to the U.S. market can create competitive advantage. Opportunities to smuggle contraband in licit commerce reflect the level and nature of trade and other economic ties between 'home' nations and the U.S. The rise of major Mexican DTOs can be explained in large part by their proximity and superior access to the U.S. cocaine market. Moreover, producer nations do have considerable domestic demand for coca, the cultivation of which exerts a locational 'pull' on cocaine refining operations.

States can either enhance or detract from the development of competitive advantage by domestic firms through their influence over the four determinants (Porter, 1990: 73). The state's impact is often subtle and occasionally unintended, arising from a wide variety of policy choices including: subsidies, product standards, labor and capital market regulations, tax policy, and antitrust laws. In the case of the cocaine trade, the most obvious and important state influence is counter-drug enforcement efforts. Because they impede the efforts of traffickers, they stimulate innovation and adaptation. While law enforcement activities may eliminate less capable actors in the drug trade, others merely refine their operations and continue operations.

A second relevant issue regarding the influence of the state is that the very existence of regulatory structures provides multinational firms the opportunity to shift activities between locations according to differentials in the regulatory surface (Dicken, 1992: 118). Operational mobility allows firms to exploit national differences in ways that create or enhance competitive advantage. Decisions to develop international strategic alliances or engage directly in overseas operations can therefore be seen, in part, as responses to regulatory differences. Lee (1999:2) notes that drug trafficking organizations routinely engage in 'regulatory arbitrage' to minimize risk and maximize efficiency. The capacity of DTOs to exploit differences in state policy and its enforcement ranks among their greatest strengths, and is a central focus in this research.

MULTINATIONAL BUSINESS STRATEGIES AND THE 'VALUE CHAIN'

Globalization has fundamentally altered the economic, political and social landscapes on which all enterprises act. The rapidly growing number of business organizations of all types pursuing multinational strategies is perhaps the most significant manifestation of these changes. Multinational strategies offer firms the opportunity to shift resources and operations across the economic landscape to exploit differences in markets, factor endowments, and government policies from place to place (Dicken, 1998; Hayter, 1997; Dunning 1993; Gray and Gray, 1981). Because globalization processes reduce the friction of economic interaction between places, they enhance the profitability of such strategies.

Criminal entrepreneurs have also implemented multinational business strategies to take advantage of opportunities provided by new economic and regulatory landscapes (Lee, 1999: 6; Castells, 1998). As their power and sophistication grew, DTOs operated outside their traditional parameters—rapidly identifying and exploiting opportunities into new geographic areas. Some major organized crime groups have expanded their operations to the global scale, while smaller criminal enterprises expand beyond their own borders to develop a regional presence (ICTA, 2000: 9).

Analysis of the organizational and spatial structure of a multinational business enterprise starts with the firm's value chain—a linked sequence of activities in which each stage adds value to the product (see Porter, 1985: 33–39). As Haig (1926: 426) noted, "every business is a package of functions and within limits these functions can be separated out and located at different places." Firms must integrate and manage this series of functional linkages across space. Those firms most efficient at the task gain competitive advantage over rivals.

The production and distribution systems of business enterprises are dynamic and must occasionally be reconfigured through the relocation or elimination of activities. Such changes are often planned strategic moves to address internal (firm) or external (industry) circumstances. They might also be hasty responses to sudden crises. Stressors include "declining demand, increased competition in domestic or foreign markets, changes in the cost or availability of production inputs, militancy and resistance of labour forces in particular places, or the pressure of national governments to modify their activities or even to cede control (Dicken, 1998: 219)." Stressors can also be positive stimuli, like the growth of new markets or the development of a new production process.

Regardless of their sources, adaptations to the organizational structure, strategic goals, or day-to-day operations of an enterprise will have specific spatial expressions. While technological advances in communications and transportation have eased the development of an integrated global economy, distance and place remain fundamental considerations. Dicken (1998: 11) notes that every firm and every component in their production chains are 'grounded' in specific locations. Multinational actors must

> configure their component parts geographically. Because different parts of the firm have different locational needs, and because these may be satisfied in different types of locations, each tends to take on distinctive geographical characteristics (Dicken, 1998: 241).

The strategies pursued by a multinational enterprise determine its 'footprint' on the landscape. Strategic choices reflect political, economic, and social characteristics of the firm's national home base, its corporate culture and administrative heritage, and the industrial environment in which it operates (Laulajainen, 1995).

Dunning's (1977) seminal explanation of multinational firm behavior also reflects the critical importance of space and place in the management of value chains. He argues that business enterprises pursue multinational strategies for three reasons: to exploit market potential; to secure raw materials; or to exploit some firm-specific competitive advantage (e.g., unique resources such as patents, trademarks, or managerial and technical skills which allow it to attain a greater degree of efficiency and increased market power). Multinational enterprises pursue competitiveness not only by exploiting some firm-specific advantage; but by doing so in conjunction with a foreign location-specific advantage (Dunning, 1997: 401).

Location specific advantages reflect spatial differences in culture, commercial practices, market conditions; barriers to trade, and the price, availability, and quality of factors of production. Such advantages are reflected in the spatial organization of production and distribution chains by DTOs. Raw materials are produced in one place, manufacturers convert raw materials into a consumable product in another, and distributors transport it to consumers in yet another. The various functions are located in those places where profits are maximized while risk is minimized.

VERTICAL INTEGRATION

An important strategic option for business enterprises is the internalization of upstream or downstream functions of the production process. Downstream (forward) integration implies the acquisition of capacity in marketing and distribution. Upstream (backward) integration internalizes functions that create inputs. By internalizing functions, an enterprise gains control over the timing and size of flows between linked stages in the value chain. Firms seek to expand internal capacity when they identify functions that can be done more efficiently than if left to imperfect external market mechanisms (Shepherd, 1997: 188).

Structural imperfections in markets (and the corresponding incentive to internalize business functions) commonly arise in industries where transaction costs are high. Transaction costs

> relate to the costs of searching for information about markets and supplies, the costs and uncertainties of negotiating contracts and the vulnerability that potentially arises from failures by independent firms in meeting the terms of contracts (Hayter, 1997: 278).

The central advantage gained by vertically integrated DTOs is the minimization of transaction costs, which are higher in the cocaine trade than in legal markets because

> advertisement cannot be used; disputes arising from differences in price, quality, service, and/or location are not necessarily settled by legal competition; and merchants do not have access to legal recourse in the case of illegal practices (Rengert, 1996: 19).

The difficulty of executing large financial transactions in an environment lacking police or courts to enforce contracts emphasizes the importance of developing reliable business 'connections.' When market participants have secure connections, business operates smoothly; without them, business operates with much higher risk (Moore, 1990: 138–39).

State policies can stimulate vertical integration by creating distortions in markets or the allocation of resources, which business enterprises either seek to exploit or protect themselves from (Dunning, 1977: 402–403). He also notes that the friction of distance may encourage internalization (Dunning, 1977: 409). Both cases are relevant to the cocaine industry, where state anti-narcotics efforts distort market mechanisms and heighten the costs and risks associated with moving the product from source to market. Criminal groups involved in the cocaine trade seek to maximize the proceeds from their participation by controlling multiple elements of the production and distribution chain. The more functions DTOs can internalize, the more they are able to limit transactions costs and improve efficiency. This 'centralization imperative' is present in most DTOs, but only the best organized and resourceful succeed in its implementation (Maingot, 1999: 150). These have developed sufficient expertise, connections, and assets to maintain an infrastructure of linked 'cells' which fulfill specific functional needs.

> Each of these subordinate functions operates in slightly different ways, recruits from different segments of society, and performs unique, yet critical functions in the overall scheme. Within each organization the division of labor is highly complex and organized (Filippone, 1994: 327).

Functional cells are rigidly compartmentalized and often managed by small tight-knit groups of relatives and friends, making them especially secure. Command and control functions are securely located in the firm's home territory, where top managers directly coordinate the actions of subordinate cells. Castells (1998: 168) notes that DTOs

> base their management and production functions in low-risk areas, where they have relative control of the institutional environment, while targeting as preferential markets those areas with the most affluent demand.

This type of structural configuration is reminiscent of the 'classic' global strategy of many licit multinational corporations, which implies tightly centralized control of assets, resources, information, and decision-making (Dicken, 1998: 204). It emphasizes geographical concentration of production at 'home,' with goods distributed to overseas markets through the firm's transportation and marketing infrastructure. This type of strategy capitalizes on centralized knowledge and scale economies, both of which are important elements in the structure of the cocaine trade. The centralization of expertise and knowledge is especially relevant, considering that excessive dissemination of knowledge and responsibility to dispersed functional 'cells' might compromise the security of the entire operation.

Vertical integration strategies allow DTOs to exploit scale economies. Major DTOs can afford to maintain in-house capacity for intelligence, communications, and security functions; are better able to manage risk and bear losses; and are better able to relocate functions away from law enforcement pressure. Just as Caves (1971: 13) described for licit firms, international expansion by DTOs involves considerable capital expenditures that bigger firms are better able to afford. The difficulty and costs involved in developing a viable multinational infrastructure constitutes another significant barrier to entry for aspiring minor DTOs.

FLEXIBLE NETWORKS

The benefits of vertical integration in the cocaine trade are real and significant. Nonetheless, fully vertically integrated trafficking organizations, like the Medellín or Cali 'cartels' of the 1980s and early 1990s, have disappeared. While such organizations have historically dominated the cocaine trade, the trend has given way in recent years to greater decentralization. Large, high-profile trafficking organizations are simply too vulnerable to law enforcement operations, while decentralized, flexible networks of smaller, specialized firms offer enhanced security by diluting law enforcement efforts (Maingot, 1999: 166). Flexible production methods can also help firms innovate and improve efficiency (Wheeler, 1998: 240). Hayter (1997: 40) notes:

> Advantages associated with specialized labor are reinforced by the advantages of specialist entrepreneurs who, motivated by self-interest, seek ways to reduce costs and / or new opportunities to define and refine market niches.

The shift from a cartel-based cocaine trade to one comprised of flexible networks mirrors recent changes in the organization of production in other industrial sectors. Throughout much of the twentieth century, 'Fordism' was the dominant production model, emphasizing internal economies and large-scale continuous flow manufacturing processes (Dicken, 1998: 165–167). This approach has slowly been replaced beginning in the late 1960s by production systems that emphasize external economies of scale and scope achieved through vertical disintegration, subcontracting, and the development of strategically interdependent networks of associated firms (Wai-Chung, 1994: 462–464).

This transition away from 'Fordist' production has been termed flexible specialization, post-Fordism, after-Fordism, or lean production (Dicken, 1998: 165; Hayter, 1997: 37). The multitude of terms used to describe this shift reflects the "strongly opposed interpretations of the nature of Fordism itself and of what it is being replaced by (Dicken, 1998: 167)." The Fordist production system was itself never as pervasive as is often claimed, with flexible, small-scale production always coexisting with mass production methods (Hayter, 1997: 38). This has certainly been the case in the cocaine trade, where small enterprises have played important roles in the industry before, during, and after the period of dominance of the Medellín and Cali cartels.

Moreover, it is difficult to identify a single distinct global trend in the organization of production that might be seen as an alternative paradigm to supplant Fordism (Dicken, 1998: 166). Business enterprises, even those operating in the same industry or industry sector, organize and manage their value chains using quite different strategies. Indeed, this very flexibility is one of the hallmarks of 'post-Fordist' production. Flexibility must exist not only in the production process itself, but also in the management of upstream and downstream linkages with associated firms. The efficient management of such networks is increasingly important, given the fragmentation of once-integrated production and distribution systems into a series of externalized functions.

The high degree of functional specialization implied by this system depends on the development of strategic alliances between internationally dispersed economic actors. Such collaborative ventures are now the core of global strategies for many multinational economic actors, allowing them to accomplish goals they could not achieve on their own. Business partnerships allowing firms to pool risk, reward, resources, and information are commonly organized through informal, interpersonal ties (Wai-Chung, 2000). The personal nature of these relationships is especially relevant in the drug trade, given the absence of legal dispute resolution mechanisms and the ever-present threat from both competitors and state authorities.

The emergence of a strikingly complex international network of business partnerships among major and minor DTOs is the most apparent manifestation of 'after-Fordism' in the cocaine trade. "By emphasizing local flexibility and international complexity, the criminal economy adapts itself to the desperate control attempts by rigid, nationally bound state institutions (Castells, 1998: 203)." In developing strategies,

> criminal organizations increasingly seek partners abroad to maximize market opportunities, improve logistics, and reduce business exposure. Often

this means relying on a foreign partner's smuggling or money laundering networks and superior knowledge of local conditions (Lee, 1999: 15).

The coordination of such networks is a challenge in any industry, but even more so when conducted in the face of mounting law enforcement pressure. Yet the success of traffickers in doing so is evident in Lee's (1999: 3) observation that the shift from a 'cartel' based structure to smaller, specialized enterprises has occurred with no noticeable decrease in the supply of cocaine. This suggests a relatively smooth introduction and implementation of flexible production methods in the drug trade.

A network approach to transnational crime reflects a growing appreciation of network organization and governance in explaining all manner of economic and social systems (see Castells, 2000; Hakansson and Johanson, 1993; Axelsson and Easton, 1992). The network is considered the basic unit of economic organization and therefore the appropriate unit of analysis for examining strategy and structure in economic systems (Hagstrom, 2000). Networks are a series of nodes (which may be individual entrepreneurs, organizations, or institutions) connected by flows of goods, services, capital, and information. Such alliances provide flexibility and allow members to pursue external economies by sharing knowledge, resources and risk. Moreover, their spatial diffusion and compartmentalized nature serve to "distance the criminal hand from the criminal mind (Passas, 2001: 30)."

Williams (2002: 73–75) argues that criminal enterprises moved at least as rapidly and thoroughly as their counterparts in licit industry to adopt flexible production and network relations. Law enforcement efforts forced them to operate covertly—focusing less on rigid structures and fixed investments and more on flexible organization and cooperation with groups that have complementary skills or resources. A good example of cooperative network relationships are the alliances that Colombian cocaine trafficking organizations formed with Italian and Russian criminal groups to facilitate distribution in European markets. Not all network interactions involve this sort of long-term cooperation, however. Many involve short-term contract relationships or even one-time exchanges of specific goods or services.

Considering that the cocaine trade is currently characterized by vertical 'disintegration,' trafficking organizations need not perform all functions of the production and distribution chain to be considered 'major' DTOs. For instance, major trafficking organizations based in Mexico and the Dominican Republic lack the capacity to produce their own product, while many major Colombian producers lack sufficient distribution capacity. Collaborative relationships with foreign traffickers allow major DTOs to subcontract various functions to specialists. These 'minor' DTOs are present throughout the production and transit zones and often perform just one function—refining, transportation, warehousing, packaging, or cross-border smuggling. Minor Mexican DTOs, for example, offer a range of services to major Colombian DTOs, particularly the direct delivery of large shipments to wholesale-level customers in the United States (USDOJ, 2001c: 4). While these local organizations lack their own distribution networks (due to high entry barriers at that stage), they are adept at cross-border smuggling or money laundering.

The flexibility and diversity of network organization reflects the dynamic nature of criminal economies themselves. Some market participants are eliminated while new entrants are attracted by high profits. State regulation and the intensity with which it is enforced varies through time and space. There may be shifts in market demand, the introduction of new sources of supply, or even new products. As industry conditions change, so do appropriate business strategies. Flexible production and network organization allow criminal actors to best respond to emerging opportunities and threats.

INNOVATION IN THE COCAINE TRADE

Expanded international business opportunities, competition, and law enforcement activities have stimulated DTOs to become more sophisticated and professional. Rather than passively accepting the effects of increasing law enforcement as inevitable, DTOs implement short- and long-term operational adaptations that minimize the effectiveness of state efforts to control the trade (Riley, 1996; Kennedy, Reuter, and Riley, 1993). When anti-narcotics measures become a hindrance, traffickers respond by developing new production techniques and marketing strategies or adjusting the combination of factor inputs required at the affected stage. Such responses might include: exploiting alternate sources of raw materials; lengthening the distribution chain; technological, process, or managerial advances that promote factor substitution and savings; or simply moving to a new location (Rasmussen and Benson, 1994).

Drug trafficking organizations routinely take advantage of commercial and technological advances in licit industries to expand and improve the efficiency of their own operations (ICTA, 2000: 9). They launder proceeds and manage finances using experienced financiers, accountants, and lawyers. They also employ transportation specialists and legal experts to research commercial flows, administrative procedures, and tariff laws in commercial ports. These professionals commonly have advanced degrees, many from prestigious U.S. universities (ICTA, 2000: 9; McCaffery, 1998b; 2; Filippone, 1994: 335).

DTOs acquire state-of the-art equipment, including encrypted communications, radio monitoring gear, night vision devices and weaponry (USDOJ, 2001: 2; Holden-Rhodes, 1997: 85). Some have developed and manufactured "super go-fast boats," with greater speed, endurance and cargo capacity than other smuggling craft (McCaffery, 1999: 5). Others have added chemical compounds to cocaine HCl to produce a substance undetectable by standard chemical tests or drug dogs (USDOJ, 1999). International partnerships between criminal organizations have facilitated these developments. For instance, linkages with Russian groups have allowed Colombian DTOs to purchase Russian military helicopters, submarines, and other gear (Acosta, 2000; Lee, 1999: 16; Maingot, 1999:145; Castells, 1998: 172).

DTOs have also successfully recruited chemists, intelligence and security personnel, and other technical specialists left under-employed after the collapse of the Soviet bloc (McCaffery, 1999: 5; McCaffery, 1998b: 2). Their intelligence units are often built around a core of former military intelligence professionals and employ a sophisticated "counter-intelligence system that identifies upcoming operations, undercover activities, and intelligence initiatives and works to thwart their effectiveness (Holden-Rhodes, 1997: 85)." Extensive networks of informants provide major DTOs with surprisingly sophisticated and useful intelligence capabilities. Mexican traffickers, for example, conduct extensive surveillance operations at U.S. border checkpoints, gathering intelligence on shift changes, traffic volume, and the diligence and effectiveness of individual officers or canine units (Brzezinski, 2002: 29). Such information is used to route shipments through the most favorable lanes and times.

The most important source of innovation and flexibility for DTOs stems from their use of location substitution strategies, popularly referred to as the "balloon effect" (Schemo and Golden, 1998). This term refers to the displacement of contained gases when compressed, and reflects the demonstrated ability of DTOs to shift operations away from those locations or routes characterized by relatively intense law enforcement efforts. As state efforts against one source or route become more effective, incentives mount to increase production, trans-shipment, or distribution in other, less risky locations (see Clawson and Lee, 1996; Caulkins, 1994; Caulkins, Crawford, and Reuter, 1993).

Perhaps the most obvious case of location substitution practiced by DTOs was the dramatic shift in smuggling routes from the Caribbean to Mexico beginning in the late 1980s (see Chapter 5). A subsequent (and equally significant) adaptation made by Colombian traffickers in the 1990s was to shorten their supply lines and increase local supplies of intermediate cocaine products (Clawson and Lee, 1996: 18). The emergence of a series of U.S. built radar installations and an aggressive air interdiction campaign raised the costs of moving inputs from Peru and Bolivia to Colombia (USDOJ, 1996b). The resulting increase in coca cultivation in Colombia has allowed local DTOs to cut costs and risk while increasing efficiency. Other cases of location substitution by DTOs occur on smaller geographic scales. For example, the Cali 'cartel' dispersed production and management operations from its home base of Valle de Cauca to other regions and countries to deter law enforcement efforts (Holden-Rhodes, 1997: 104).

Innovation is a critical component in the development of competitive advantage by business enterprises. Any stressor that interferes with the sustainable profitability of an organization can generate an adaptive response. The most obvious stimuli include competition, state regulation, or a change in the availability or price of factors of production. Regardless of its source, innovation often results from organizational learning rather than a formal process of research and development (Porter, 1990: 45). 'Learned' innovative responses to stressors are common in the cocaine trade, and help explain the long-term success of both individual DTOs and the industry as a whole.

PRICE STRUCTURE

The term price structure refers to the amount of value added at each stage of an industry's production and distribution chain. In the cocaine business, both the magnitude of value added and some of its sources differ from licit industries. The most striking characteristic of the price structure of cocaine is the astonishing scale of value added during the production and distribution process. Approximately 350 kg of leaf, worth about $400, is refined to produce one kg of cocaine HCl (hydrochloride), worth perhaps $100,000 or more at the retail level. Former director of the Office of National Drug Control Policy, Barry McCaffery, commented:

> Drug syndicates wield a powerful instrument for subverting even relatively strong societies: a money machine. Like modern-day Midases, they transform an intrinsically cheap and available commodity into an almost inconceivably remunerative product. . . . They (drugs) are relatively cheap to produce and offer enormous profit margins that allow the drug trade to generate criminal revenues on a scale without historic precedent (McCaffery, 1998b: 5)."

Of course, McCaffery's "money machine" is a fiction. In fact, drug prohibition is the mechanism that transforms coca from cheap commodity to immensely valuable consumer product. Drug enforcement can be modeled as a tax that raises the supply curve and leads to higher equilibrium prices and greater spending on drugs (MacCoun and Caulkins, 1996: 186). Caulkins (1994b: 10) notes, "increasing interdiction increases the quantity and value of drug exports, thereby increasing revenues for drug suppliers in the source country."

For any product, the price paid by consumers is the sum of all production and distribution costs. These commonly include raw materials, services, capital goods, and wages. Prices for both cocaine HCl and intermediary products are relatively volatile, reflecting a number of influences: law enforcement efforts, market competition, changing consumer preferences, and advancements in the manufacturing process. Producer costs in cocaine manufacturing include coca leaves, precursor chemicals, and processing equipment. Coca leaves are very inexpensive, accounting for less than one percent of the retail price of cocaine. The required chemicals have many licit industrial uses and are readily available. Antezana (1996) estimates that production costs in the base extraction stage are roughly $540 per kilogram. This includes $420 for coca leaf and $120 per kilogram for precursor chemicals and labor. Even in the final stage of refining, where the required chemicals are more expensive and often must be imported, procurement costs account for only a small fraction of the retail price of cocaine (Riley, 1996: 82).

Table 2.1 Cocaine Industry Approximate Price Structure

350 kg coca leaf—Bolivia	$400
1 kg cocaine base—Bolivia	$600
1 kg cocaine HCl—Colombia	$1,200
1 kg HCl–Guatemala	$2,500
1 kg HCl–bulk wholesale (Reynosa, Mexico)	$6,000
1 kg HCl—bulk wholesale (McAllen, TX)	$10,000
1 kg HCl—bulk wholesale (Chicago)	$18,000
1 kg HCl—downstream wholesale (Chicago)	$24,000
1 kg HCl—bulk retail (ounce)	$35,000
1 kg HCl—retail (gram dose)	$90,000

Sources: Economist, 2001d: 6; National Drug Intelligence Center, 2001: 2; National Institute on Drug Abuse, 2000: 29–30; ONDCP 2000a: 71 and b: 20, USDOJ, 1998; Holden-Rhodes, 1997; Antezana, 1996; personal communication.

The transportation of cocaine from producer countries to the U.S. is a notable source of added value. Management of the trans-shipment process is complicated and involves numerous costs: aircraft or maritime vessels, pilots, maintenance and landing rights; loading, unloading, packing, storage, transaction costs, security, intelligence collection, and bribes. Corruption functions as an informal 'tax' on smuggling and traffickers viewed it as a necessary business expense (Andreas, 1999b: 92).

Value added for cocaine at each stage is also a function of the amount of risk present at that stage (Economist, 2001d: 6). Risk and value added increase as the product moves toward the distribution stages, in a manner that does not necessarily correspond to factor opportunity costs. Paste, base, and HCl are more valuable than leaf and more likely to be the focus of law enforcement efforts. A more significant increase in prices (and revenue) can be identified in the industry's downstream activities—smuggling, wholesale distribution, and retailing. In these stages, attendant risks are much higher. While risk premiums are indeed significant, they do not by themselves account for huge increases in value added for cocaine. Explanations that over-emphasize risk and under-emphasize tangible, out-of-pocket costs like transportation and security are deficient.

The distribution of income earned at various stages of the production process varies dramatically as well. Distribution is wide spread at the cultivation stage, but becmes increasingly concentrated through the manufacturing

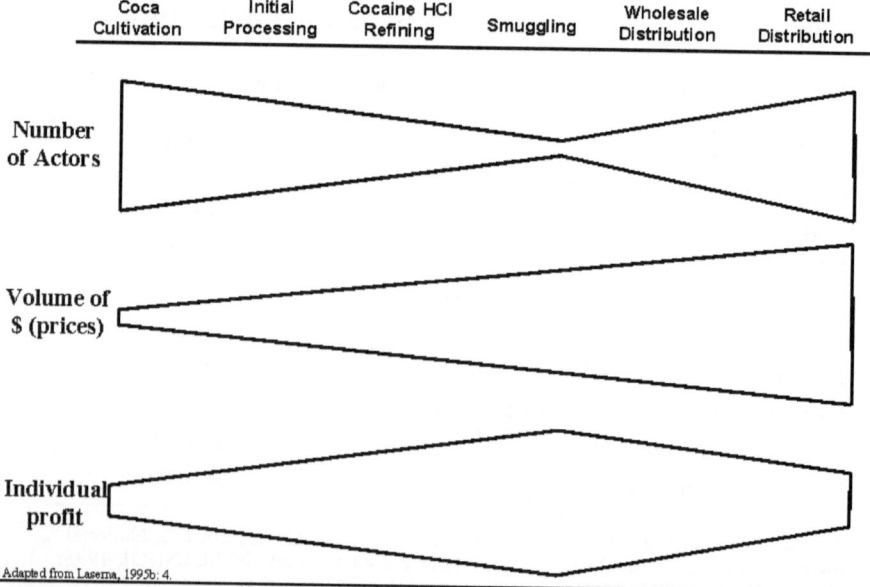

Adapted from Laserna, 1995b: 4.

Figure 2.1 Income Distribution

stages. Income becomes gradually more broadly distributed as one follows the distribution network downstream. At the retail level, income distribution again becomes widespread.

This chapter builds a conceptual foundation regarding the spatial organization of the cocaine industry and its component firms. Subsequent chapters will develop a more complete and detailed understanding of the operations of DTOs at various stages of their value chain. The case study chapters illuminate local manifestations of the global processes involved. These differences are best explained by examining of the confluence of unique local environments and economic and political trends at the global scale. It is to this task that the research now turns.

Chapter Three
From Coca to Cocaine

The cultivation and use of coca in the Andes dates back more than four thousand years. Coca leaves were an important element in the social and religious organization of the region's pre-Colombian civilizations (Laserna 1995b: 45; Erickson, 1994: 5). It was (and remains today) an important element in the diets of indigenous highlanders, serving to suppress hunger, relieve altitude sickness and provide supplemental nutrition (Morales, 1992: 165). In the mid 16th century, Spanish traveler Pedro Cieza de Leon noted:

> The Indians carry this Coca in their mouths; from morning until they lie down to sleep they never take it out. When I asked some of these Indians why they carried these leaves in their mouths, which they do not eat, but merely hold between their teeth, they replied that it prevents them from feeling hungry, and gives them great vigor and strength (in Mortimer, 1901).

The Spanish originally restricted the use of coca, but acquiesced when they realized its capacity to stimulate and sustain indigenous laborers (Erickson, 1994: 5; Mortimer, 1901). Leaf production in colonial times was concentrated in Bolivia's Yungas region, already established as a major production center under the Incas (Klein, 1992:277). Growing demand from mining districts in the *altiplano* stimulated an expansion of cultivation under Spanish rule.

> So vital was this consumption that coca leaf often served in place of money wages and was the most highly commercialized Indian product in the colonial Andean world, sometimes serving as money in even Spanish commercial exchanges (Klein, 1986: 23).

Today, coca remains a powerful cultural icon for indigenous Andean populations. Bolivian presidential candidate Evo Morales recently called it "our new national flag" (Padgett, 2002). Coca and coca products such as

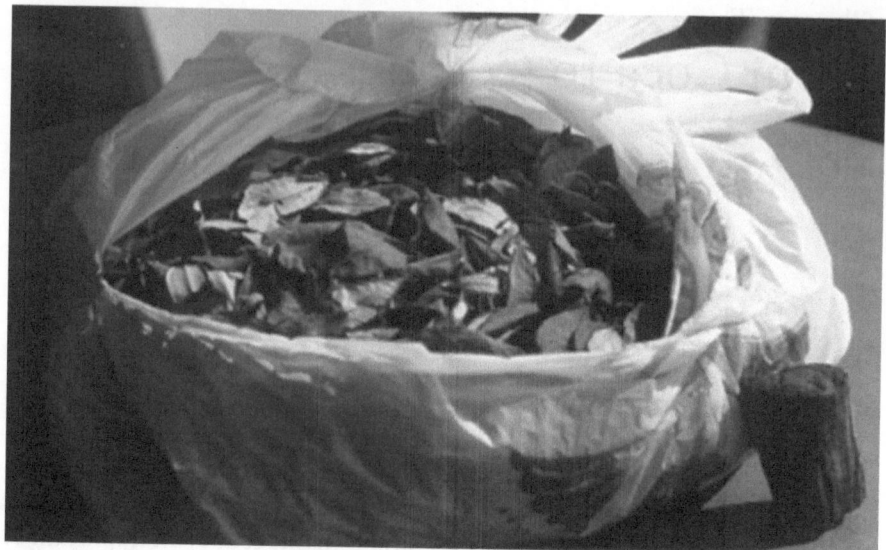

One pound of coca leaf used for chewing. Next to the bag is a chunk of legia, chewed with a mouthful of leaves to help release the cocaine alkaloid.

tea and medicines are sold openly and used for a variety of purposes, especially the alleviation of fatigue and the effects of altitude. Laserna (1995b: 56) argues that ninety percent of rural Bolivians regularly consume coca in one form or another. The tough and adaptable bush is also an important and relatively profitable element of Andean agricultural systems. Coca flourishes on steep slopes and in poor soils that hinder the growth of other crops. It also tolerates a wide range of altitudes, climatic conditions, and is more resistant to disease and insects than other cash crops. Correspondingly, coca can be grown almost anywhere in tropical South America (Clawson, 1996: 131).

Coca yields two to six harvests a year, depending on the particular strain and local growing conditions. Annual yield estimates per hectare range from 1.8 to 7.6 metric tons of leaf (Antezana, 1996; Sanabria, 1993: 44–45). These differences can be explained by the presence of differently aged plants within fields, inter-cropping, soil type, the number of harvests, and seasonal variations. Coca cultivation is by a wide margin the most labor-intensive stage in the value chain of the cocaine trade. Farmers must first grow or acquire seedlings, then build terraces or burn and clear forest. Once seedlings are planted and fertilized, they require occasional weeding, pruning, and (depending on availability) periodic applications of pesticide (Sanabria, 1993: 44). The bushes must mature for at least 18 months before the first crop can be harvested, and full production is not reached for two to

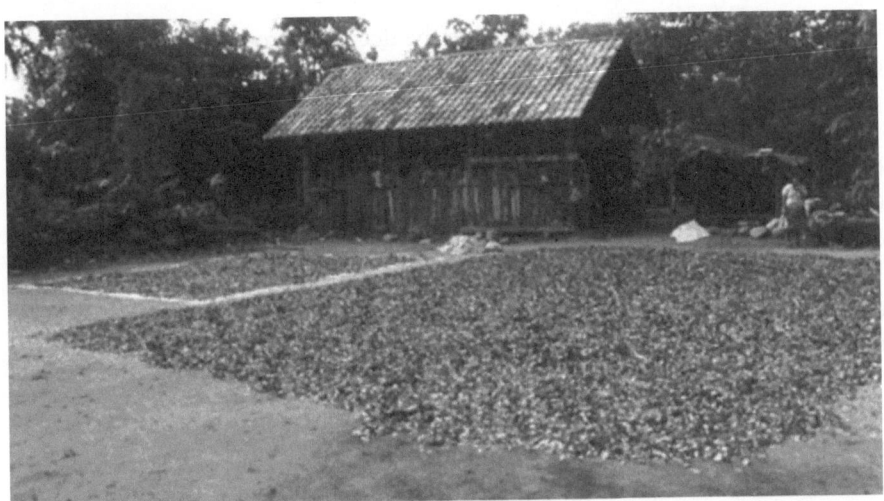

Coca leaves drying before processing in Chapare, Bolivia.

four years. After harvesting, leaves must be dried in the sun within two to three days or they will mildew. They are then transported to market or paste processing locations in hundred pound bundles known as *cargas* (Riley, 1996: 78).

Coca cultivation requires only rudimentary tools and minimal capital investment. Production costs (excluding labor) for cultivating coca are roughly $170 annually per hectare (Antezana, 1996). These include land preparation, equipment, coca seedlings, rental value of the land, and agro-chemicals. These factors make coca an attractive cash crop for un- and under-employed peasant laborers abundant throughout the Andean region. Traditionally, coca has been grown primarily in small, peasant owned farms in Bolivia and Peru (Klein, 1992: 277). The typical family farm might grow one or two hectares of coca inter-cropped with five to seven acres of subsistence crops (Clawson, 1996: 132). A hectare plot would produce about 3 metric tons of leaf per year, enough raw material for roughly 7–8 kg of cocaine (Antezana, 1996).

Coca cultivation is concentrated in two regions of Bolivia—the highland Yungas and lowland Chapare. It is more widespread in Peru, with major concentrations in the Huallaga and Apurimac valleys. (Figure 3.2) In the mid-1990s, these regions accounted for about three-quarters (164,000 hectares) of all coca cultivation. By 1999, however, U.S authorities claimed that eradication campaigns had reduced the regions' share to about one-third (61,000 hectares) of total cultivation (INCSR: 1999). Observers suggest, however, that official figures overstate the decline in coca cultivation in both countries (Economist, 2000d: 23). Production there has likely been displaced to more remote sites rather than eliminated.

Over the same period, coca cultivation increased dramatically in Colombia, from 51,000 Ha to 123,000 Ha (INCSR: 1999). It is now widespread in Colombia, with significant concentrations in the plains and tropical regions of the remote southeastern departments of Meta, Guaviare, Vaupes, Caqueta, and Putamayo (Menzel, 1996: 8). Coca cultivation continues to expand in Colombia, with the UN Drug Control Program estimating that more than 400,000 Ha were dedicated to coca in Colombia by 2001 (Forero, 2001). A sharp recent decline in coffee prices has created a 'coffee crisis' throughout the Andes, exacerbating a more general economic downturn (Economist, 2001d). As unemployment grows and coffee's prospects dim, peasant farmers have begun to replace coffee plants with coca (Wilson, 2001). Meanwhile, coca leaf prices are rising throughout the region, further increasing the opportunity costs paid by farmers tending alterative crops (Hall, 2000).

Drug trafficking organizations have chosen not to be directly involved at this stage. This decision reflects the relatively insignificant costs of coca inputs compared to downstream costs and profits. Moreover, large-scale operations for growing or refining coca in cultivation areas are relatively easy targets for state anti-drug operations. The absence of large-scale coca 'plantations' in most growing regions can be seen as a strategy of the trafficking elite to shift risks to peasant farmers (Sanabria, 1993: 14). A notable exception

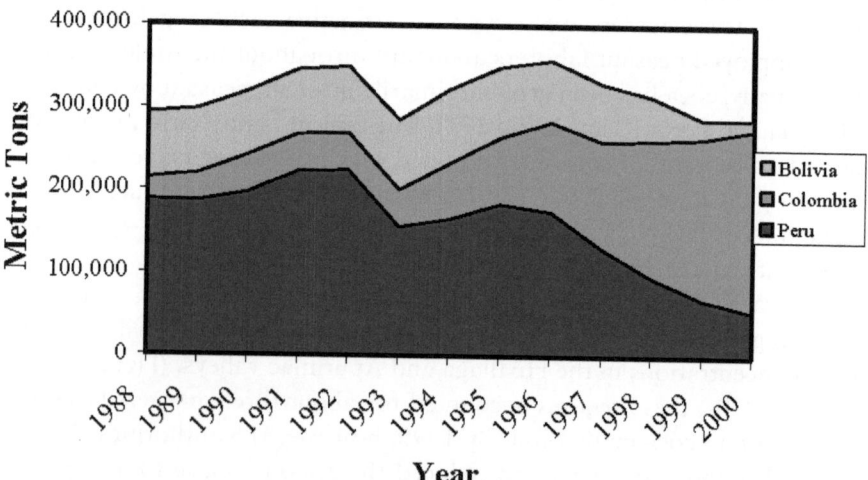

Figure 3.1 Coca Leaf Production, 1988–2000

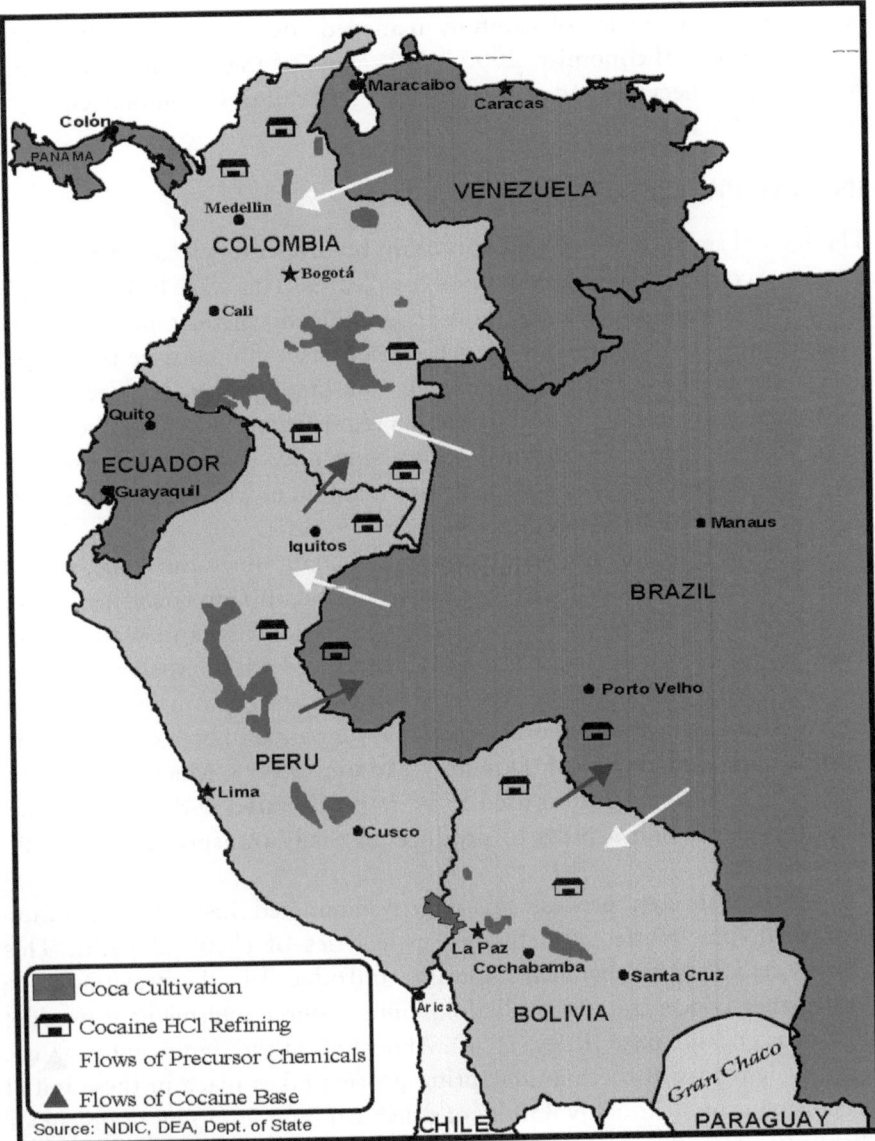

Figure 3.2 Andean Production Zone

is the recent emergence of carefully managed coca plantations in remote rural Colombia (Economist, 2000d: 23). Most of these plantations range from 10 to 80 hectares and now supply roughly half of Colombian coca leaf (UNDCP, 2001b).

INITIAL PROCESSING

The second stage of the production chain involves the release and concentration of cocaine alkaloid from dried coca leaves. This stage has historically encompassed two functionally and geographically distinct processes: the production of coca paste and the refining of paste into cocaine base. Over the last decade, however, a more efficient "one-step" process has become the norm, especially in Bolivia and Colombia (Antezana, 1996). The coca paste stage was eliminated, with initial processing now using an intermediary known as *agua rica* (a suspended cocaine alkaloid in weak acid solution) to produce base (Holden-Rhodes, 1997: 159).

The first steps of the refining process remain much the same, requiring a maceration pit lined with cement or plastic, mixing containers, basic drying and filtering equipment, a variety of chemicals, and water. Dried leaves are placed in the maceration pit and treated with kerosene and a series of alkaline and acidic solutions. The leaves are vigorously stomped in each mixture by peasant laborers known as *pisacocas* to break down the alkaloids contained in the leaf (Dombrey-Moore, 1994: 8; MacGregor, 1993: 105). The resulting solution used to be re-precipitated with soda or lime, then passed through a press to produce an easily transportable, grayish-white paste.

In the 'one-step' process, this stage is eliminated. Instead, the solution is washed, precipitated and filtered in a series of chemical baths. This process removes the chemical impurities introduced in the previous stage and further concentrates the alkaloids into a purer intermediate product known as cocaine base (Riley, 1996). Almost all of the significant raw material weight loss in the manufacturing process takes place in these initial processing stages. Roughly 350 kg of dried leaf (and 30-40 kg of precursor chemicals) are needed to produce 1 kg of cocaine base (Antezana, 1996; Riley, 1996; Dombrey-Moore, 1994). The bulk of large quantities of coca leaf, and the fact that they lose much of their weight during initial processing, means that paste and base processing facilities tend to locate near coca sources. The large quantities of water required for initial processing mean that these operations must also be oriented toward water sources. Once leaves are processed into cocaine base, however, it is easily transported and can be further refined almost anywhere.

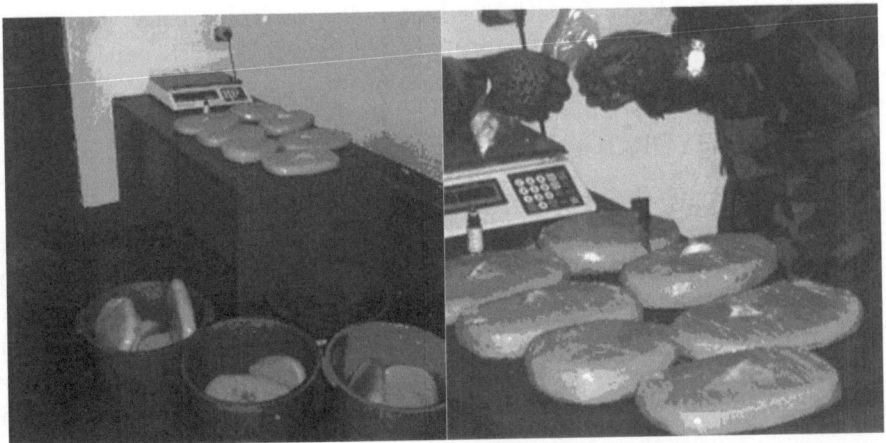

80 kg of cocaine base seized in the Chapare, Bolivia. Each solid 'brick' weighs about 1kg.

Skilled labor requirements for initial processing stages are minimal, requiring just a basic knowledge of the proper mix of chemicals. Adequate manual labor for mixing, stomping, and packaging are also necessary. These laborers are closely linked to coca farmers, both socially and geographically. Because the process is not very complicated, peasant farmers and laborers have been enticed into base production as a way to maintain income levels as coca leaf prices have declined. The result has been a dramatic growth of simple, small-scale processing facilities in Andean cultivation areas (Healy, 1994: 205).

Initial refining processes are characterized by diseconomies of scale because large operations are tempting targets for law enforcement. DTOs realized that it was more convenient for growers to make paste or base in small, dispersed facilities—they are easier to construct and conceal than large centralized operations. Typical peasant operators might produce a few kilograms at a time and sell them to trafficking groups, which transport the coca base to well hidden and defended facilities for further processing into cocaine HCl (Riley, 1996: 79).

Throughout the 1980s and early 1990s, there was a great deal of cross-border trade in intermediary coca products. Bolivian and Peruvian paste and base were routinely transported to Colombia for further refining (Kennedy, 1993: 43; Dombrey-Moore, 1994: 12). By the mid 1990s, however, most domestically grown coca leaves were processed into base in-country (USDOJ, 1996b, Clawson and Lee, 1996: 151). There were two main factors influencing this shift. First, aggressive air interdiction efforts dramatically increased the risks involved, particularly for high-bulk, low-value paste shipments. Second, 'local' DTOs and farmers expanded their productive capacity over time, in an effort to maintain or increase profits.

COCAINE HYDROCHLORIDE

The final step in the refining process transforms base into cocaine hydrochloride, the purest and most marketable form of the product. Cocaine HCl is an odorless crystalline powder classified as a central nervous system stimulant. The alkaloid was first isolated and named by German scientist Albert Niemann in 1860. Researchers were soon investigating its medicinal potential. Among these early studies was Sigmund Freud's 1884 work *Uber Coca*, in which he commented "I have tested this effect of coca, which

Table 3.1 Potential Cocaine Base Production (mt), by Growing Region

		1996	1997	1998	1999
Guaviare	Colombia	187	141	130	136
W. Caqueta	Colombia	52	79	92	62
E. Caqueta	Colombia	42	58	80	86
Norte de Santander	Colombia	0	0	11	32
San Lucas	Colombia	0	0	12	17
Arayca	Colombia	0	0	0	5
Putamayo	Colombia	26	70	111	169
Macarena	Colombia	0	0	0	9
Upper Huallaga Valley	Peru	141	121	99	69
Central Huallaga Valley	Peru	18	9	4	2
Lower Huallaga Valley	Peru	15	8	3	2
Aguaytia	Peru	59	32	18	8
Pachitea	Peru	31	11	6	4
Apurimac	Peru	104	83	56	37
Cusco	Peru	18	15	13	11
Other	Peru	22	18	13	10
Chapare	Bolivia	142	128	82	10
Yungas/Apolo	Bolivia	30	31	29	18
Total		887	803	759	687

Source: ONDCP, 2000.

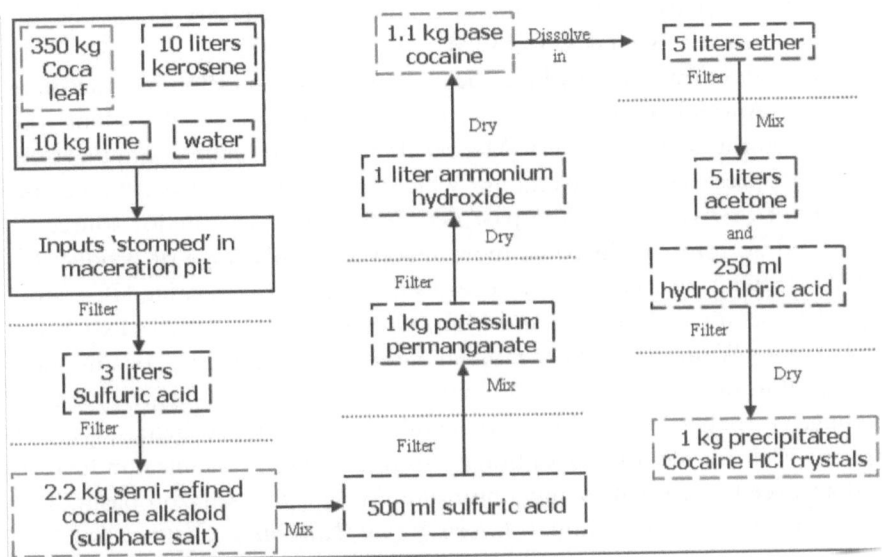

Figure 3.3 Cocaine HCl Production Chain

wards off hunger, sleep and fatigue and steels oneself to intellectual effort (in Erickson, et. al., 1994: 8)." Yet the use of cocaine as a local anesthetic and for other medical applications was insignificant relative to its commercial exploitation. Pharmaceutical firms and other manufacturers marketed a wide variety of cocaine products, including inhalers, creams, cigarettes, and dozens of varieties of wines and soft drinks (Laserna, 1995b: 78–79). Their irresponsible promotion, commercial success, and the abuses that resulted eventually led to the prohibition of coca and cocaine products.

The terminal refining process that produces cocaine HCl is relatively sophisticated, requiring technical expertise, capital investment in equipment, and a skilled work force. In this stage, cocaine base is dissolved in ether and mixed with hydrochloric acid. It is then cooked, dried, and filtered into pure cocaine HCl. Very little weight reduction takes place during this transformation (Dombrey-Moore, 1994: 8; Riley, 1996: 80). Traffickers have historically looked to exploit economies of scale in production at this stage. Sophisticated and well-guarded laboratories concealed in remote locations are designed to process up to twenty tons of cocaine HCl per month. Refining facilities can employ as many as one hundred and fifty workers and include communications centers, generators, chemical recycling facilities, living quarters, recreational facilities, airstrips, and warehouses in addition to the lab itself (Clawson, 1996: 38). DTOs often maintain excess laboratory facilities, so in the event that a lab or two are shut down, processing capacity will not be significantly reduced (Kennedy, 1993: 44).

Labs have traditionally been located on ranches in Colombia's desolate *llanos* in Antioquia and Cordoba, or in the remote jungles along the Peruvian and Brazilian borders (Menzel, 1997: 9). The state maintains only a minimal presence in these regions, which are isolated by dense jungle and a network or rivers. Over the past decade Brazil, long a major source of ether and acetone, has become more involved in this stage of production (OGD, 1996: 176; Clawson and Lee: 1996: 232). Now cocaine HCl refining labs operate in Rondonia and Mato Grosso, states in Brazil's expansive and remote Western frontier (Holden-Rhodes, 1997: 115). Cocaine base produced in Bolivia and Peru is commonly exported to this region for processing. Traffickers here exploit two significant advantages: better access to precursor chemicals (thanks to Brazil's sizable domestic chemical industry); and an excellent riverine smuggling route through the Amazon basin. The Department of State's annual *International Narcotics Control Strategy Report* (2000) estimates cocaine production (in metric tons), by country for the three major producers:

	Colombia	Peru	Bolivia	Total
1999	520	175	70	765
1998	345	240	150	825
1997	350	325	200	875
1996	300	435	215	950
1995	230	460	240	930
1994	70	435	255	760
1993	65	410	240	715
1992	60	550	225	835

Such figures are over-simplifications based on estimates of coca cultivation and conversion (refining) rates. They fail to reflect the reality that Colombia has always dominated the production of cocaine HCl. These numbers are better indications of how much coca leaf or base was produced rather than the amount of cocaine hydrochloride. The *potential* might have existed for Peru and Bolivia to produce hundreds of tons of cocaine HCl in the early to mid 1990s, but this potential was never realized. Colombian DTOs have historically purchased the majority of cocaine intermediaries produced in those two countries and transported them to Colombia for final processing. In Bolivia and Peru, the focus of the cocaine trade has traditionally been on coca cultivation and the early stages of processing. These 'national' roles have blurred in recent years, as Colombia emerged as the top coca producer, while Bolivian and Peruvian DTOs expanded their cocaine smuggling and distribution networks. Despite this convergence, there remain noteworthy differences in the nature of the cocaine business in each. The following case study of the historical development of the coca-cocaine industry in Bolivia illuminates such differences.

COCA-COCAINE: THE BOLIVIAN CONTEXT

Bolivia entered its worst economic crisis in a century in the mid to late 1970s. The collapse resulted from a combination of falling commodity prices (especially in mining), huge debt-service payments, and government mismanagement (Laserna, 1995b: 38–43; Klein, 1992: 271–272). Bolivia's Gross Domestic Product declined by more than two percent a year from 1981 to 1986, and barely kept pace with population growth until 1991. Real wages and living standards declined dramatically during this period, and the official unemployment rate (usually a gross underestimate) topped twenty percent, while inflation reached more than 8,000 percent (Painter, 1994: 6; Morales, 1993: 159).

Economic crises have lasting effects on social, economic and political institutions and commonly precipitate economic displacement, new industrial systems, and new geographies of competition (Glasmeier, 2000: 23). Bolivia's 'lost decade' was no different, for it had substantial implications for Bolivia's fragile economy and civil society. As the crisis deepened, a concurrent rise in international demand for cocaine created powerful incentives for Bolivian entrepreneurs, state officials, and peasants to enter the trade (Morales, 1992: 161). In Bolivia's case, the link between economic crisis and drug trafficking is readily apparent—cocaine offered a means of economic survival in difficult times for all (Laserna, 1995b: 20).

Economic development programs funded by international lenders in the 1960s and 1970s gave rise to a powerful agribusiness and ranching elite concentrated in Santa Cruz and Beni departments. The collapse of world commodities markets in the 1970s stimulated these desperate entrepreneurs to develop the country's coca-cocaine industry (Holden-Rhodes, 1997: 44; Malamud-Goti, 1992: 70). As profits from licit activities fell, the processing and smuggling of coca-cocaine products expanded. As the industry grew, traffickers consolidated sufficient economic and political power to protect themselves from Bolivia's weak central government (Sanabria, 1993: 58).

Successful organizations were close-knit, family-based enterprises with close ties to like-minded elites and to Bolivian police and military authorities. They also enjoyed stable and diverse connections to international criminal networks, and played surprisingly important roles in the pan-American cocaine trade in its early years. Gamarra (1999: 172) notes, "as early as 1978, Bolivian organizations were able to deliver refined cocaine to distribution networks on both the East and West coasts of the United States." During this early period, the Santa Ana 'cartel' emerged. It was a major, fully vertically integrated DTO headquartered in Beni department that would dominate the Bolivian industry for more than a decade (Gamarra, 1999: 176–183). The enterprise linked a network of coca cultivators and maceration pits located throughout the Chapare with refining labs in Beni using a fleet of small aircraft. The group also developed an in-house capacity for international transportation, wholesale distribution and money laundering.

Most Bolivian DTOs did not achieve the same degree of sophistication. The typical Bolivian trafficker still processed leaves into paste (and later base), then sold it to Colombian buyers for further processing. By the mid 1980s, a few other Bolivian DTOs had diversified their operations and markets, in an effort to capture the higher profits found in the downstream stages of production and distribution (Healy, 1994: 205). These groups developed internal capacity for cocaine HCl production and some successfully developed small-scale distribution networks. As Bolivian coca cultivation expanded, refining, storage, and transportation facilities appeared throughout the remote stretches of Santa Cruz, Beni, and Pando departments. Hundreds of rudimentary airstrips scattered throughout the region facilitated the movement of intermediary products and supplies throughout Bolivia and the rest of Andean South America (Painter, 1994: 24).

Meanwhile, downstream refining operations in Colombian were characterized by excess productive capacity. Domestic access to cocaine intermediaries was limited at the time, stimulating a few Colombian DTOs to expand operations to Bolivia. Their Bolivian operations enjoyed stable local access to coca inputs, and major trafficking centers managed by Colombian DTOs soon emerged in Huanchaca (Santa Cruz) and La Floresta, Santa Ana, San Ramón, and San Joaquín (Beni). All were remote and inaccessible, close to the Brazilian border, and populated by independent residents long neglected by the state (Painter, 1994: 28–30).

The profits of local Bolivian traffickers were squeezed by competition from more efficient and better-connected Colombian groups. They responded by gradually adopting technologies and business practices from their Colombian partners and rivals. To exploit economies of scale, they

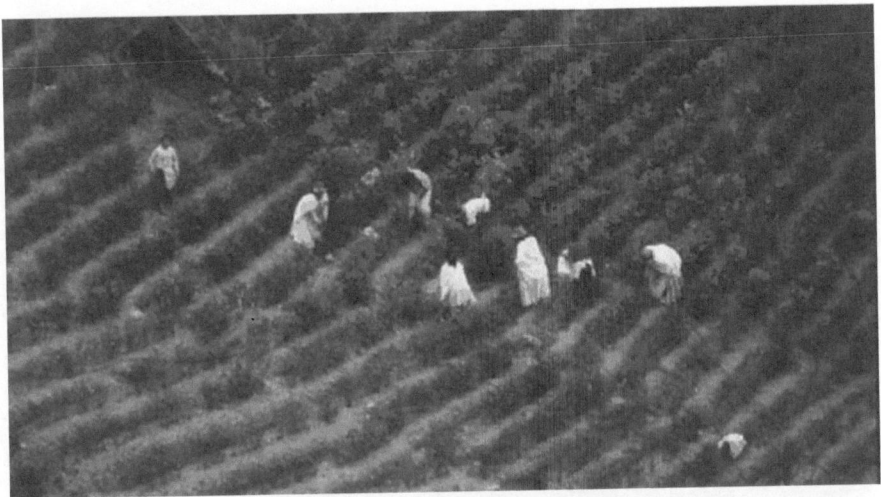

Women harvesting coca leaves on a terraced hillside outside Chulumani, Yungas.

vertically integrated operations, from paste purchases to processing to smuggling. Less profitable initial paste processing operations were left to farmers. By 1990, there were perhaps two-dozen domestic DTOs involved in the coca-cocaine industry in Bolivia. Together, they processed about a third of Bolivian-made paste into 150 to 200 tons of cocaine HCl within Bolivia (Painter, 1994: 28). By the mid 1990s, roughly half of Bolivian-grown coca leaf was refined into cocaine HCl in-country (Clawson, 1996: 13).

Despite their growing productive capacity, most Bolivian DTOs were not capable of full independence from their Colombian associates. While a few major trafficking groups managed to establish profitable distribution networks using Mexican and Brazilian partners, the majority still concentrated on production rather than distribution. Bolivia's geographical and economic isolation, shortage of capital, and lack of smuggling connections and marketing expertise mean that most domestic groups continue to sell the majority of their product (whether base or HCl) to Colombian DTOs for distribution.

Just as drug trafficking provided opportunities for Bolivia's elite, coca cultivation did the same for the country's impoverished peasantry. Bolivia has historically produced about a third of the world's coca leaf, though its share has declined in recent years due to aggressive U.S.-backed eradication efforts (USDOS, 2000). It is grown here in two main regions—the *Yungas* is the traditional center of cultivation and the area from which licit coca is supplied to the domestic market. The terrain there is rugged (with elevations

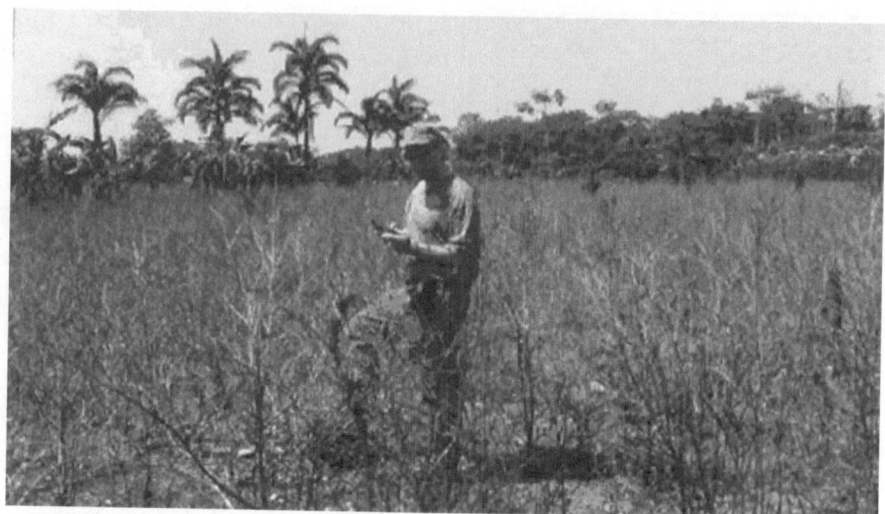

The author in a recently harvested coca field east of Chimoré, Bolivia.

ranging from 1,000 to 8,000 feet), making road building and mechanized agriculture difficult (MacGregor, 1993: 3). Peasant farmers here tend relatively large communal coca fields planted on terraced mountainsides.

The Chapare region is comprised of lowland subtropical rainforest east of and parallel to the eastern slopes of the Andes. The terrain is characterized by dense vegetation and acidic and nutrient-poor soils. After the forest is cleared, heavy seasonal precipitation washes away the relatively small amount of organic matter in the soil, and yields of many crops are rapidly reduced (MacGregor, 1993: 4). The average peasant farm in Chapare has from 2–4 hectares under cultivation at any one time, roughly a third of which is dedicated to coca. The rest is cropped with bananas, cassava, corn, citrus fruits, and other minor crops. The variety of leaf grown in the Chapare has less alkaloid content and an off taste, making is less favored for traditional uses. Not surprisingly, most of the coca grown here is intended for cocaine refining.

The Chapare occupies roughly half the land area of Cochabamba, Bolivia's most densely populated department. Two-thirds of Cochabamba's population is rural farmers in highland villages, where population pressures and land fragmentation have resulted in a widespread system of tiny, inefficient landholdings called *minifundios* (Sanabria, 1993: 21). The Bolivian government has failed to implement meaningful land reform or resolve income disparities in these impoverished and volatile highland communities. The state has instead sought to ease social pressures by using the country's

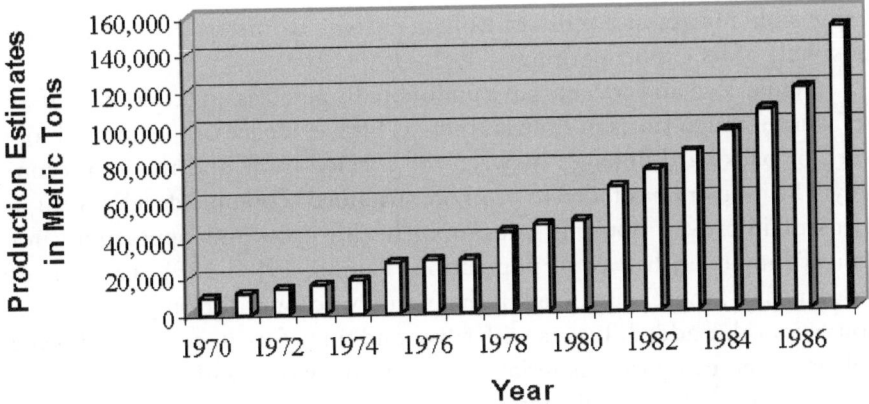

Figure 3.4 Bolivia's Coca Boom

undeveloped eastern lowlands as a 'safety valve'. Attempts to encourage migration to the lowlands allow for the transfer of lands from the government to individuals willing to relocate from highland communities (Sanabria, 1993: 42).

As of the late 1960s, there were about 25,000 residents in the Chapare. A decade later, its population reached about 80,000, and by the end of the 1980s, had jumped to more than 200,000 (Painter, 1994: 4). Coca was well suited to absorb the thousands of landless highland peasants pouring into the region, and its cultivation increased dramatically beginning in the late 1970s. It soon eclipsed production in the traditionally dominant Yungas, and by the end of the 1980s accounted for perhaps ninety percent of Bolivia's total output (Sanabria, 1993: 59). Despite this growth in population and activity, the region remained poorly connected to the rest of the country—its isolation encouraging the continued cultivation and initial processing of coca.

The coca-cocaine industry has provided a number of benefits to Bolivia's economy in the form of employment, income for peasant farmers, and export earnings. These benefits were of particular importance during Bolivia's 'lost decade,' when coca was its only major source of economic growth (Klein, 1992: 279). Estimates from the 1990s suggest that from 74,000 to 500,000 Bolivians were employed in the cultivation, processing, and transportation of coca and cocaine intermediaries (Gamarra, 1999: 172; Clawson, 1996: 15; Painter, 1994: 40; Morales, 1992: 137). Considering that the economically active population of Bolivia in 1990 was only 1.8 million, the industry was clearly a major source of employment regardless of which estimate is used. During this period, it was also responsible for about a tenth of Bolivia's Gross Domestic Product and al-most half of its export earnings (Healy, 1994: 205).

While coca and cocaine have undoubtedly acted as an economic 'safety net' during tough times in Bolivia, there is little evidence of meaningful for-ward or backward linkages between the cocaine trade and the legal econ-omy. The industry has failed to promote sustained economic development in terms of improved housing, education, health care, and opportunity for Bolivia's impoverished rural population (Painter, 1994: 139). The tens of thousands of laborers involved in the industry account for only a tiny frac-tion of its value added. Just as with silver and tin before it, coca has allowed Bolivia to serve as a raw material supplier to the world without its realizing the industry's full economic potential. Moreover, its potential in Bolivia has diminished for the time being, as U.S. backed eradication campaigns have curtailed coca cultivation. Such success has been accompanied, however, by serious social and economic costs, including deepening poverty, unemploy-ment, and civil unrest (Economist, 2001a; Cabrera, 2000; Krauss, 2000). The industry remains a strong presence in Bolivia and eradication efforts will generate continued social, economic, and political disruption.

CONTROLLING COCA

The primary U.S. effort to disrupt the cocaine trade has been to reduce coca cultivation by making it less appealing to peasant farmers. The methods used to accomplish this goal have been forced and voluntary eradication, and alternative development programs, especially crop substitution. Despite a significant commitment of resources, the task of eliminating coca has been a difficult struggle with little tangible long-term success at the regional (Andean) scale. While there have been short-term and local successes, these accomplishments provide little reason for optimism regarding the broader program. To appreciate the challenging nature of eradication efforts, it is im-portant to understand the appeal of coca to the region's farmers.

- Coca can reach maturity within two years of planting, faster than most other cash crops. It enjoys a relatively long productive lifes-pan and requires less attention and investment than other crops once it has been planted.
- Once harvested and dried, leaves spoil relatively slowly and are not subject to damage during transport. These are major advan-tages in cultivation regions characterized by grossly deficient transportation infrastructures.

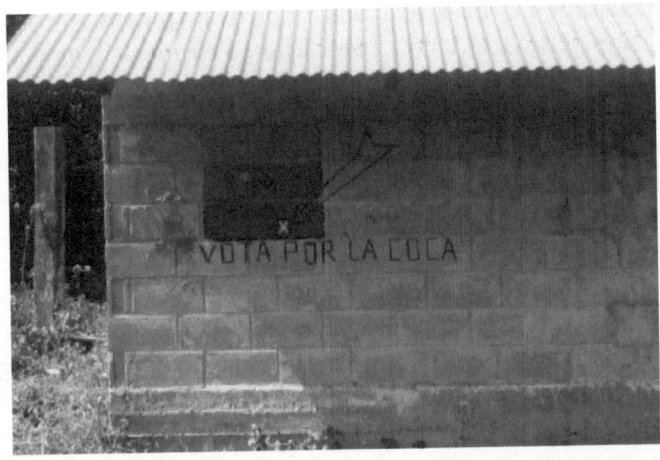

Storefront in a small, rural commercial center near Chimoré, Bolivia.

- Peasant farmers are familiar with coca and the skills necessary for cultivating it.
- Coca can provide up to six harvests a year in a region where most crops give one. More importantly, it has access to a guaranteed local market, providing year round income and insurance against unusual weather-related or other disasters.
- It is highly adaptable to many climates and conditions and can be grown in bad or depleted soils. It can replace other crops that have exhausted the soil or expand the agricultural frontier into land not otherwise suitable for farming.

Coca plants are considered the most visible and vulnerable element of the production chain by counter-drug authorities. Plants are fixed assets, immobile in the short-term, and subject to relatively easy detection and elimination. Moreover, the longest lag in the production chain is at the cultivation stage. Farmers need a minimum of two years to locate new land, re-plant and wait until they can reap their first harvest.

In Bolivia, the U.S. has pursued coca eradication goals using both forced and voluntary programs. Until 1998, the most common approach was voluntary eradication, which compensated farmers for destroying their own crops. Despite U.S. skepticism of the approach, it has traditionally been favored by the Bolivian government. Democratic institutions are weak there and the state has been reluctant to provoke potentially disruptive elements in society (Riley, 1996: 136). The government feared that forced eradication would generate conflict with Bolivia's unions, especially the politically powerful coca growers. Concerns also emerged that the repressive treatment of farmers, combined with an absence of income alternatives, might stimulate the development of guerilla movements like those in Peru or Colombia (Lee, 1999: 5).

Voluntary eradication programs have had little success, however, in reducing coca cultivation in Bolivia—it remained stable at about 55,000 ha throughout much of the 1990s (INCSR, 1997: 71). Its failure is not surprising, considering a basic limitation of voluntary eradication programs. As farmers turn in their crops for compensation, a smaller amount of coca is produced. Yet the demand for cocaine (and thus coca) remains unchanged. In time, coca prices rise to ensure that enough is produced to meet demand. Eventually, the price offered for coca will top that offered for voluntary eradication, and farmers will be enticed into cultivation once again. The $2,000 compensatory payment per eradicated hectare has actually served as a minimum price, preventing farmers from having to absorb the full effects of price reductions brought about by interdiction (Healy, 1994: 210; Painter, 1994: 89). Worse, farmers have moved into more remote areas to plant new fields after receiving the compensation payment, often in exchange for older bushes whose productive life was coming to a close anyway (Riley, 1996: 210).

The limitations of voluntary eradication programs precipitated a major shift in U.S. policy in Bolivia in 1998. Beginning late that year, U.S. coordinated and supported forcible eradication efforts targeted all coca fields outside traditional, legal growing areas (basically the Yungas) for destruction without compensation to the farmer. The Bolivian military had been conducting similar operations since 1991, but mounting U.S. frustration with the pace and efficacy of this program eventually forced its expansion and intensification. With this shift, social tensions in Bolivia and especially the Chapare have escalated into a series of protests, riots, strikes and violent confrontations between armed eradication teams and local peasant groups (Economist, 2001a,c; Flaherty 2001: 25; Cabrera, 2000). Repressive measures aimed at coca farmers have generated widespread discontentment and opposition, yet Bolivia's dependence on foreign aid leaves it subject to U.S. demands regarding anti-drug strategies.

It is not clear that forced eradication efforts will restrict coca cultivation in the long-term anyway. Rather, it displaces existing coca farming to more remote places where eradication pressure is less intense (Laserna,

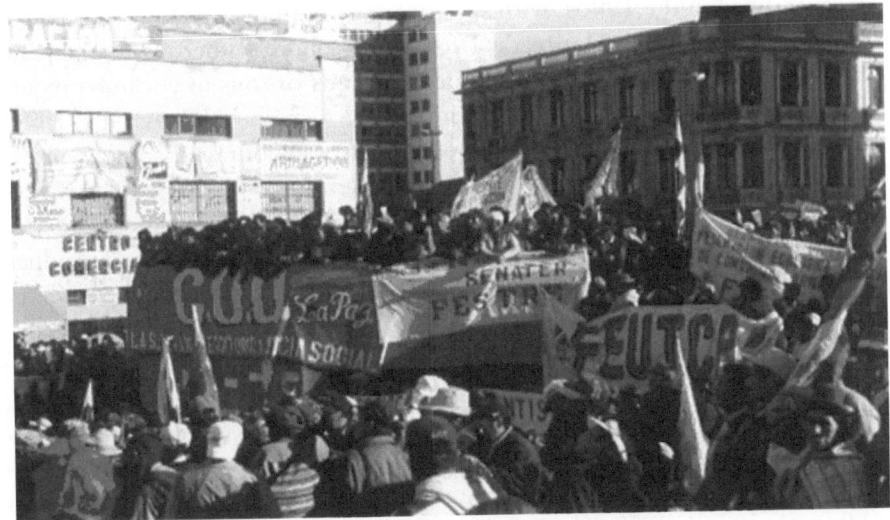

A 1998 protest against U.S. backed forced eradication programs. Coca growers from across the country marched to La Paz to register their concerns regarding the end of voluntary (paid) eradication.

1995b: 28). Location substitution by farmers is facilitated by both the abundance of suitable alternative locations in Andean South America, and by the lack of state control over vast swathes of the region's territory. Kennedy (1993, 5) suggests that coca is currently cultivated on less than one percent of the land in which it might potentially be grown. Riley (1996: 142) notes that there are perhaps 40 million hectares that could potentially host coca cultivation in Bolivia and Peru.

In many ways, the cocaine industry has developed in Peru as it has in Bolivia. Until the mid-1990s, Peru was the leading producer of coca leaf and paste. At this time, the coca-cocaine industry accounted for about four percent of GDP and employed anywhere from 175,000 to 300,000 people (Clawson, 1996: 15 and Riley, 1996: 137). Since 1996, coca cultivation in Peru has declined steadily; the result of aggressive, U.S. backed eradication and air interdiction campaigns. By late 2000, however, coca prices in Peru had risen sufficiently to induce peasant farmers to return to the crop (Guggenheim, 2000). Factors in the resurgence of coca prices include greater demand for inputs from Bolivian traffickers, and the anticipation of supply disruptions in Colombian coca production areas as a result of Plan Colombia (Chapter Four).

Coca cultivation and processing has traditionally been located in the Huallaga valley on the Eastern slopes of the Andes. The industry has decentralized in the 1990s, with significant growth in Amazon regions like Apurimac, Aguaytia, Madre de Dios, and Puno. Numerous clandestine landing strips there are used to export hundreds of tons of cocaine precursors to Colombia annually for refining into cocaine HCl (OGD, 1996: 162). Effective air interdiction campaigns have encouraged some well organized Peruvian DTOs to develop downstream capacity in cocaine HCl refining, smuggling, and distribution. While these firms seek independence from their Colombian counterparts, most of the cocaine HCl they produce is still sold to Colombian buyers for distribution through traditional channels (USDOJ, 1996b).

ALTERNATIVE DEVELOPMENT

The success of coca eradication schemes (if they can be successful at all) depends upon the cooperation of source countries. While the perceived vulnerability of the cocaine trade at the cultivation stage makes it appealing to U.S. anti-narcotics officials, it is less obvious why source countries would want to control cultivation. Coca has extended the agricultural frontier, relieved land pressures, and provided foreign earnings and employment benefits. The importance of the coca-cocaine industry to the region is linked to long-term poverty and under-development. Hundreds of thousands of impoverished and landless peasants have moved to take advantage of the opportunities offered by coca. In these countries, the industry is less a law enforcement problem than a development problem that requires development-oriented solutions.

Alternative development programs supported by the U.S. are managed by U.S. Aid for International Development and seek to identify other sources of income for peasant farmers. The major alternative development effort undertaken by USAID in Bolivia has been the Chapare Regional Development Project (CRDP), begun in 1983. Its focus has been to assist farmers to substitute other cash crops for coca and (later) to develop processing and packaging facilities for local produce. The program has been limited since its inception, however, by insufficient funding, policy changes, corruption, bureaucratic rivalries, and the lack of a clear strategy (Painter, 1994: 108).

The remoteness of peasant plots, bad weather, and a deficient transportation infrastructure create other problems. Farmers must pay very high transportation costs to move produce to market. These costs comprise perhaps eighty percent of the value of products exported from the Chapare (Clawson, 1996: 148). The markets for most alternative crops are far enough away to make transporting them uneconomical. Therefore, most crops can only be sold in the local market, which would diminish if the coca industry were eliminated. Many alternative crops are highly perishable, and the lack of local processing facilities makes it difficult to regularly supply a stable amount of exportable crops. For this reason purchasers are reluctant to place orders without assurance that they will be filled, and farmers are reluctant to plant unless they are assured of markets.

An important element of the Chapare Regional Development Project is a pair of agricultural research and extension centers, supported through U.S. Aid for International Development, at La Jota and Chipiriri. The program has identified a number of crops considered viable alternatives to coca, including: macadamia nuts, coconuts, black pepper, dyes, and various fruits. Local farmers have criticized the program, however, for focusing on theoretical on-site research while failing to help farmers identify and resolve problems on their own plots. Worse, the program has been production-driven, rather than market-driven. It has been undeniably successful in determining the technical viability of certain crops and the physical conditions and inputs required to maximize their production. Where it has not succeeded is in identifying where and how these crops will be processed or sold (Painter, 1994: 118). Holden-Rhodes (1997: 172) notes:

> The continuing dilemma of income replacement is the issue of getting crops—any crops—to market. Coca is contracted for, paid for, and picked up by the narcotraficantes, thus ensuring a completed production cycle that puts money in the hands of the campesino. Any crop that is recommended a worthy substitute has to meet the test of ability to get to market; this in itself is the very heart of the core/periphery issue in Latin America.

Coca cultivation takes place in what might be considered the periphery of the periphery. Coca growers commonly operate in the most inaccessible and lawless regions of countries which are themselves isolated from global markets and the international political community. Even if this isolation were overcome and alternative crops developed and successfully marketed, this successes might have little impact on the cocaine trade. Traffickers can match any increased economic opportunity that results from crop substitution programs. By increasing the price paid for leaves to a level above that paid for alternative crops, they can entice peasant farmers back into coca cultivation. Considering the minimal cost of coca inputs relative to costs and revenues elsewhere in their value chains, traffickers can afford to spend much more on coca without diminishing their profitability. Even exceptionally successful crop substitution programs could not counter the rising opportunity costs faced by farmers in the long-term.

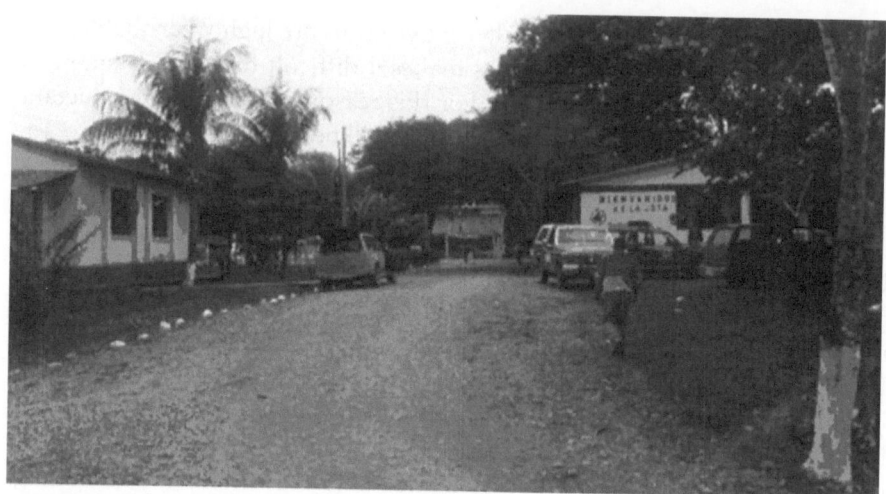

USAID supported agricultural research and extension station in La Jota, Chapare.

Despite their failures, alternative development schemes have not fared so poorly that they deserve to be dismissed entirely. They should instead be strengthened, expanded and given more time to succeed. The search for alternative sources of income in Bolivia is exceedingly difficult, considering its physical and economic isolation and the poor condition of its infrastructure. While the search may yet prove a failure, it would be ill advised to give up, especially considering the consequences of doing nothing. The development of suitable income alternatives is an important component in long-term efforts to restrict coca cultivation and helps mitigate social pressures associated with forced eradication measures.

A basic objective of this research is to demonstrate how the cocaine trade develops in different forms in different places. Local characteristics influence the functional orientation, organization, and competitiveness of local drug trafficking organizations. Variations in relevant local conditions between the three major producer countries are reflected in their respective traditional 'national roles' in the coca/cocaine trade. These roles are constructed through the interaction of 'global' processes like market oriented economic reform and the demand for cocaine and 'local' characteristics like (in Bolivia) a history of coca cultivation and use, geographical isolation, large indigenous population, extreme poverty, and unstable government. 'Local' characteristics in Colombia are not quite the same—the differences explain the unique functional orientation of the industry there, as well as its influence on the country's economic and political landscape.

Chapter Four
Colombian Competitive Advantage in Cocaine

Colombia has been involved in the international cocaine trade since the 1950s, when domestic producers supplied small quantities to organized criminal enterprises in Cuba. When the Cuban groups were displaced to Miami in the 1960s, they began to distribute small amounts of Colombian cocaine through South Florida. Meanwhile, Colombian marijuana traffickers saw a decline in the profitability of their operations due to intensified U.S. interdiction efforts. Some viewed this development as an opportunity to adapt existing smuggling networks to distribute cocaine, which was soon to experience a dramatic rise in popularity in the United States (Riley, 1996: 11).

By the mid to late 1970s, Colombian DTOs were using small private aircraft to smuggle relatively large shipments of cocaine into Florida from the Bahamas. Colombian traffickers quickly eliminated their Cuban competitors and installed their own distribution networks (Filippone, 1994: 324–325). Since the cocaine boom of the 1970s, Colombian DTOs have remained the world's largest producers and distributors of cocaine. This chapter investigates the organization and operations of Colombian trafficking groups. It also identifies and evaluates the location factors favoring the development of internationally competitive DTOs in Colombia.

The Colombian coca-cocaine industry is a networked system linking the specialized functions of the production and distribution processes. Linkages are coordinated through a complex network of partnerships and contracts among scores of minor DTOs and roughly a dozen major DTOs. The former provide all sorts of specialized services including supplies of inputs, refining, storage and transportation. Clawson and Lee (1996: 19) estimate that they employ perhaps 20,000 'specialists' responsible for handling many of the day-to-day operations of the industry. These include pilots, chemists, shippers, overseas distributors, spies, accountants, guards, couriers, and other skilled laborers.

The export-oriented, core trafficking organizations are comprised of top leaders, management, and their staffs. These enterprises manage the industry's 'flexible network' that connects the hundreds of thousands of farmers who cultivate coca and perform the initial processing of leaves with retail distribution networks at the other end of the distribution chain. Colombian entrepreneurs have achieved and maintained competitive advantage in the industry by (moving early to) develop efficient, tightly controlled brokerage services that fill this gap between peasant producers and consumers.

Their development required considerable long-term investments in transportation, communications, and security infrastructure (Riley, 1996: 172). Complex intelligence gathering and bribery arrangements were incorporated into smuggling networks to provide control over and security of shipments (Holden-Rhodes, 1997). Such arrangements smooth the flow of cocaine through or around potential choke points in the transit zone through early warning of impending law enforcement activities. The international dispersal of operations makes the development and maintenance of such infrastructure difficult and costly. They represent a significant barrier to entry for potential competitors.

Major DTOs also developed a tightly organized international marketing structure. Huge downstream revenues served as a powerful incentive for Colombian DTOs to extend distribution networks towards the retail market. They built wholesale distribution channels in the U.S. managed by marketing 'cells' staffed with salaried employees (Clawson and Lee, 1996: 39). Cell leaders reported directly to the home office, where group managers set prices, determined the volume to be sold, and approved buyers (USDOJ, 2001c; Lee, 1999: 18). Downstream marketing operations are examined in greater detail in Chapter Six.

AGGLOMERATION AND 'CARTELS'

In late 1981, Martha Nieves de Ochoa, a member of a prominent Medellín family, was kidnapped by leftist guerillas. While kidnap and ransom were (and are) commonplace in Colombia, this particular event held great significance for the cocaine trade. The Ochoa brothers were leading cocaine traffickers in Medellín, and like their peers, were staunchly pro-Colombian nationalists. They convinced dozens of Medellín-based minor and major DTOs to pool their resources to create *Muerte a Secuestradores* (MAS–or Death to Kidnappers), a paramilitary unit to fight against the leftists (Filippone, 1994: 325). Each organization contributed millions of dollars to maintain the unit, which quickly demonstrated its ruthless efficiency in winning Ochoa's release.

> Their two-thousand man hit squad rained horror and destruction on the Marxists. In Medellin, they invaded homes and blew away people merely suspected of involvement with the kidnappers . . . guerilla sympathizers were abducted and tortured. On February 17, 1982, Marta Nieves Ochoa was released unharmed (Gray, 1998: 120).

The kidnapping and its well-coordinated, brutal response were the catalyst for the development of the Medellín 'cartel.' This group was not a cartel in the traditionally defined economic sense, but rather an allied group of independent family-based trafficking organizations located in relatively close proximity to one another. While there was no formal, hierarchical form of leadership that synchronized activities, prominent leaders did emerge in coordinating roles (Lee, 1999: 19). Members expanded their early cooperation into a variety of business related functions. By coordinating trafficking activities and sharing resources, they developed an enormous pooled capacity for cocaine refining, transportation, distribution, security, intelligence, and financial management. At its peak, the organizations comprising the 'cartel' employed 120,000 people, including two or three thousand in the United States (Filippone, 1994: 324).

A crackdown by Colombian law enforcement authorities on the Medellín cartel's high profile leadership in the early 1990s had little long-term effect on the Colombian cocaine trade. The group's dominant role in the business was immediately filled by the Cali 'cartel,' which had been collaborating with law enforcement efforts targeting their competitors. In fact, Cali assassins played a major role in their rivals' downfall by killing hundreds of professional associates and family members of the Medellín leadership (Bowden, 2001). As they strengthened their grip on the cocaine trade in the early to mid 1990s, the U.S. market share of the Cali group jumped from twenty to eighty percent (Drexler, 1997: 161). Cali's annual profits at the time were estimated at $8 billion (DEA, 1996b: 3). Much like its predecessor and rival, the Cali 'cartel' was a loose regional coalition of exporting organizations, this one emerging from the Valle de Cauca area. It was comprised of a few major core organizations and dozens of smaller associated groups (Clawson and Lee, 1996: 55).

It is hardly surprising that dominant cocaine trafficking organizations would emerge in Medellín and Cali, which are Colombia's traditional entrepreneurial centers. In the 1970s, the collapse of the textile industry in Antioquia (Medellín) and the sugar industry in Valle de Cauca (Cali) helped stimulate their development as major cocaine trafficking centers (Castells, 1998: 198). Colombia's rugged Andean topography has historically magnified regional separation and association (Economist, 2001b: 5; Blouet and Blouet, 1993: 334). For this reason, Colombian DTOs commonly associate and cooperate with like-minded organizations in their home regions (Holden-Rhodes, 1997: 49). Local clusters

> co-financed and co-insured large shipments of cocaine, pooled information on law enforcement activities, developed joint counterintelligence and counter-enforcement strategies, and collaborated to improve the bargaining positions vis-à-vis the state (Lee, 1999: 18).

Such agglomerations are common in industries throughout the world and provide local firms with valuable economies of scale (Porter, 1990). Localization economies encompass a wide variety of benefits accruing to individual firms from their proximity to clusters of related activities. Foremost among these economies are the presence of a variety of service providers that supply highly specialized services and additional productive capacity in response to demand from clustered client firms (Hayter, 1997: 92). Firms also benefit by learning from 'knowledge spillovers' in relationships with partners and rivals regarding innovation and best practices in the industry. Dicken (1998: 167), Wheeler (1998: 238) and Wai-Chung (1994: 474) argue that these localization tendencies are very strong in flexible production networks due to distance decay effects on inter-firm communication and exchange. In the Colombian cocaine trade, these networks are densest in Antioquia and Valle de Cauca, home to dozens of major and minor DTOs, many specializing in relevant producer services.

Regional associations by trafficking enterprises greatly facilitated large volume smuggling. 'Cartel' arrangements were designed to maximize export volumes while minimizing risks to individual suppliers. Major DTOs initiated transport insurance programs, in which suppliers paid the insurer/shipper a small portion of the U.S. wholesale price of their shipment. If lost or seized, the insurer would replace it at the Colombian purchase price (Bowden, 2001: 24). Major exporters could make significant profits by smuggling cocaine into the U.S. for smaller operators and insuring them against loss. The importance of such arrangements should not be underestimated, considering that individual shipments might be worth of tens of millions of dollars (Riley, 1996: 173). Partnerships not only helped define the 'cartel' structure of the Colombian drug trade, but were used to attract legitimate investors to the business by offering them high returns with moderate risk. In this manner, it served to minimize the distinction between the traditional business elite and the underworld in Colombia (Bowden, 2001: 25; Clawson and Lee, 1996: 38).

After the Cali group was dismantled in the mid to late 1990s, the 'cartel' structure of the industry declined. In its place emerged a more decentralized flexible network incorporating greater numbers of smaller and more specialized DTOs. These firms remain concentrated in the Valle de Cauca region and the Caribbean north Coast, suggesting that the importance of local partnerships has not diminished (USDOJ, 2001: 4; USDOJ, 2000: 39). These organizations are still commonly run by family groups and are often closely tied to paramilitary formations (Economist, 2001b: 9). They have more expertise, capital, and better distribution networks than emerging rivals in Peru or Bolivia. Moreover, thanks to dramatic recent increases in coca cultivation in Colombia, they are no longer dependent on foreign supplies of cocaine intermediaries. U.S. anti-narcotics intelligence authorities note:

> This new generation of Colombian trafficking groups maintains lower profiles, focuses on limited aspects of the drug trade, and forms more ad hoc alliances that make them more difficult law enforcement targets (ICTA, 2000: 109).

LOCATION SPECIFIC ADVANTAGES

Over the last three decades, Colombia has offered a set of conditions that have minimized the risks of involvement in the cocaine trade, attracted the refining process, and allowed Colombians to control Andean coca markets. Dominant DTOs have continued to emerge in Colombia because of a unique combination of local characteristics that together provide domestic traffickers with significant competitive advantages. These location-specific advantages derive from a variety of sources.

The simplest and most common explanation for Colombia's success in the cocaine trade is its favorable physical location. The country is near major coca-producing regions, but closer to the U.S. market. This explanation fails, however, to take into account the exceptionally high value of cocaine relative to its volume and weight. For this reason, transportation costs (at least in a neoclassical cost-minimization sense—see Hayter, 1997: 112–115) are relatively unimportant considerations in determining the location of cocaine refining. Given the footloose nature of the refining process, such activities could just as easily be located in other producer countries. For cocaine, the physical distance between sources of supply and the market are less important than the 'economic distance'—measured in the depth of trade and financial linkages between source and destination countries. Colombian economic ties to the U.S are deeper and more diverse than those of other

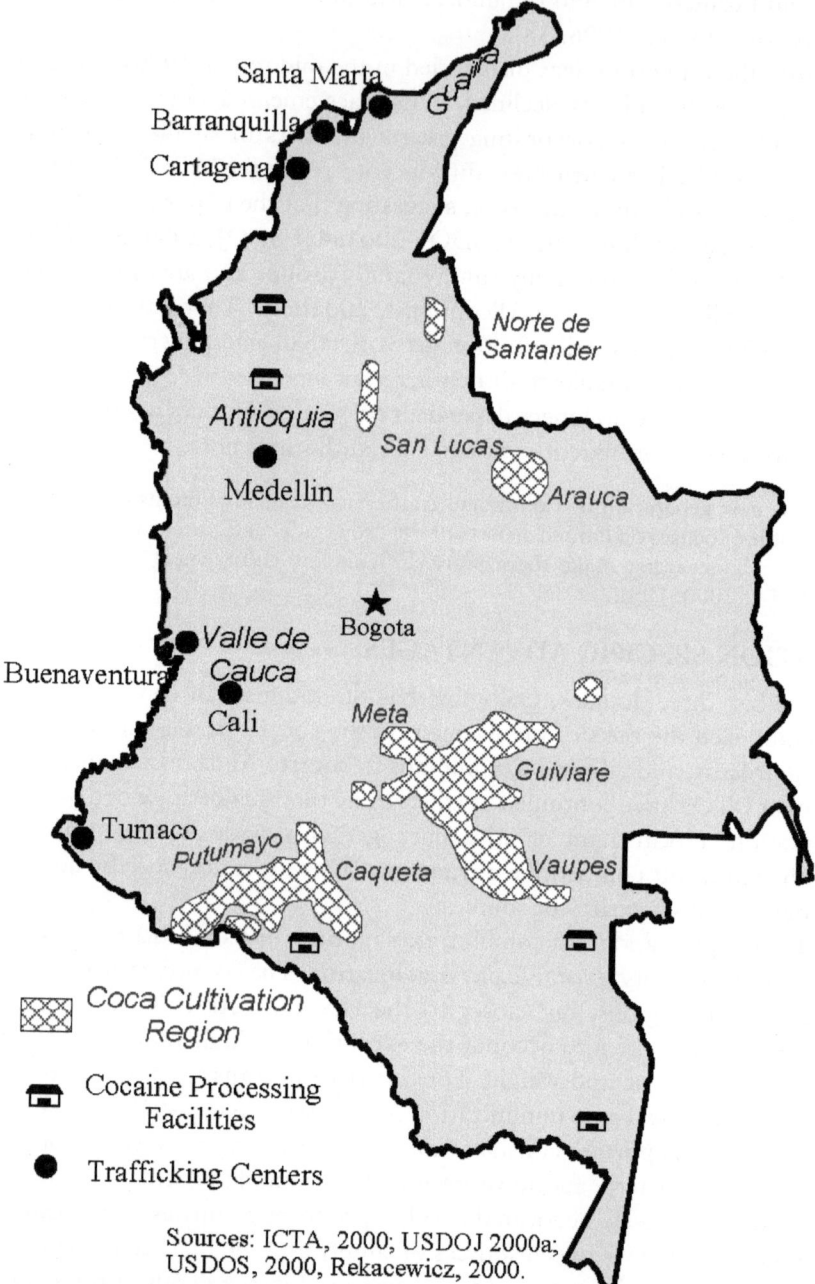

Figure 4.1 Colombia's Coca-Cocaine Trade

producer countries, providing more opportunities for successfully conceal-ing illicit transactions within licit flows (USDOC, 2002).

Furthermore, the argument explaining Colombia's advantage as the 'most accessible' location ignores that fact that Colombian trafficking groups have *created* competitive advantage in the cocaine trade by master-ing the appropriate technology and techniques required for success. Their ability to thwart enforcement efforts through bribery, intimidation, and vi-olence, as well as the ability to mobilize the economic surplus from their ac-tivities are important factors. To fully appreciate the core position of Colombian DTOs is to understand the 'local' characteristics that contribute to the development of their competitive advantage. A number of relevant factors might be cited: widespread corruption; a large informal economy; re-mote mountain and rainforest regions that facilitate the concealment of the industry's facilities; and chronic under-employment. Yet these factors are also present in other Andean nations, some with clear historical advantages in coca production. As such, they fail to identify Colombia as a uniquely ad-vantageous site for cocaine production and distribution. While each of these location factors do indeed 'attract' the cocaine trade, they fail to provide a satisfying explanation as to why Colombia occupies a core position.

A more satisfying explanation is the prevalence and widespread ac-ceptance of contraband and a long smuggling tradition (Menzel, 1997: 5). By the 1950s, the import of contraband consumer goods was institutional-ized, lending an aura of legitimacy to smuggling and diminishing any social stigma that might have been attached to it. More unique is Colombia's his-tory of exporting contraband. Livestock, coffee, and emeralds have long been smuggled from the country as a way of avoiding taxes, quotas, and other regulations. The contraband trade established linkages between Colombian and foreign smugglers, while high import tariffs and strict for-eign exchange controls encouraged an active black market in foreign ex-change. Both developments provided expertise on money laundering and developed channels for the repatriation of drug profits.

Another contributing factor is the peculiar nature of capitalism in Colombia. Colombian entrepreneurs have historically operated on the expec-tation of high short-term profits. Physical barriers to internal transportation, especially the three Andean cordilleras, have greatly segmented Colombia's in-ternal markets, causing widely differing prices. These differences spurred the rise of an entrepreneurial elite focused on trade and speculative activities, and unaccustomed to making long-term, productive investments (Thoumi, 1995: 88). This 'get-rich-quick' mentality facilitated the development and accept-ance of drug trafficking. A final important factor is the sizable population of

Colombian nationals living in the U.S. These migrants provided a labor pool from which to recruit and organize distribution networks (Menzel, 1997: 6).

This unique combination of factors has created an 'incubator' environment where Colombian DTOs have created and maintained competitive advantages. While other Latin American and Caribbean nations display one or more of these conditions, none has re-created the entire package of factors experienced in Colombia. Peru and Bolivia have come closest to replicating Colombian developments and processes, but in many cases they occurred much later. The delay gave Colombian traffickers the opportunity to establish manufacturing and distribution networks that have proven difficult to replace.

LA VIOLENCIA AND SUBSEQUENT CIVIL CONFLICT

During the 20th century, Colombia evolved quickly from a traditional rural society to an industrially based urban economy. This challenging transformation created a need for social institutions that might mitigate the stresses which accompanied these sweeping socio-economic changes. Colombian society has generally failed to meet these demands–an institutional crisis that has contributed to the country's long history of civil and political violence (Thoumi, 1995: 84). From 1948 to 1957, an undeclared civil conflict known as *La Violencia* raged throughout Colombia, killing a quarter of a million people (Clawson, 2000: 123). The struggle matched supporters of the country's two historically dominant political parties and is infamous throughout Latin America for its extraordinary levels of violence and cruelty (Watson, 2000: 531).

This unenviable tradition is reflected in the willingness of Colombian DTOs to employ violence in pursuit of business goals (Castells, 1998: 200; Menzel, 1997: 5). Terroristic violence in Colombia is both an art form and an important method of psychological warfare (Bowden, 2001: 14). The infamous 'Colombian necktie' is a signature form of this type of brutality. While deplorable in most contexts, a lack of regard for human life comes in handy in a high-profit, risky, intensely competitive industry like cocaine. The focused application of violence as a business strategy was especially prevalent during the early stages of the industry's development in the 1970s. Colombian traffickers ruthlessly eliminated their emerging counterparts in Bolivia and Peru, gaining firm control over the industry (Thoumi, 1995: 86). This head start over business rivals allowed Colombia-based DTOs to establish productive capacity, secure distribution and intelligence networks, and create nearly insurmountable barriers to entry for potential market entrants.

La Violencia ended with a power-sharing agreement between the Conservatives and the Liberals that served to de-legitimize electoral competition and the multiparty system (Economist, 2001b: 5). Guerilla insurgencies appeared as leftist political minorities found themselves left out of public affairs (Ferrerya and Segura, 2000: 24). Over time, state institutions became more inefficient and less responsive to the public. Corruption and disregard for the law grew in both public and private sectors and an underground economy flourished. The increasing gap between the rule of law and actual behavior eventually de-legitimized the state, a process considered "Colombia's main advantage as a locus for illegal drug production (Thoumi, 1995: 84)."

An especially relevant aspect of this de-legitimation was the loss of state control over large areas of the countryside. Since *la Violencia* , leftist guerillas, especially the Fuerzas Armadas Revolucionarias Colombianas (FARC) and the Ejercito de Liberacion Nacional (ELN) have controlled significant portions of rural Colombia. The regional separations imposed by three Andean mountain chains, their associated river valleys, and dense rainforests have long weakened the territorial control of the Colombian state. Even today, the central government cannot provide basic services and infrastructure in Colombia's extensive rural areas (Watson, 2000: 530). Transportation of goods and people in Colombia's 'peripheral' interior also remain difficult and costly. In the state's absence, coca plantations, refining facilities, warehouses, and airstrips have flourished, concealed by the country's sheer size and its rugged, isolating topography.

Private armies, supported by landowners, drug traffickers and the military, have emerged to counter guerilla formations in rural areas (Bowden, 2001: 33). Paramilitary formations are notorious for kidnapping, torturing, and killing non-combatant peasants thought to have leftist connections (Economist: 2001b: 3; Watson, 2000: 538). The savage conflict between these groups has accelerated over the past decade, claiming tens of thousands of Colombian lives (Ferrerya and Segura, 2000: 28). Both sides now support themselves primarily through their involvement in the drug trade.

There are about one hundred paramilitary outfits, the majority organized under the *Autodefensas Unidas de Colombia* (Economist, 2001b: 11–12; Ferrerya and Segura, 2000: 28). The AUC supports roughly three-quarters of its estimated 8,000 troops with drug proceeds (ICTA, 2000: 106; Economist, 2000g: 39). This operating capital is generated either directly through cocaine refining operations or indirectly by contributions from drug traffickers (Economist, 2001b: 24; Acosta, 2000; Sequera, 2000). The FARC is the most important and powerful guerilla movement, with roughly 12,000 regular troops. Both the FARC and ELN support themselves primarily by taxing and protecting peasant coca growers and paste processors (Economist, 2000d: 24).

Estimates of total annual drug related earnings for Colombia's guerillas range from $250 million to $500 million (Economist, 2001b; Lee, 1999:
8; Robinson, 1998). Some view these figures as evidence that the leftist insurgents have emerged as a new 'cartel,' a reaction commonly expressed as
justification for heightened U.S. military involvement in Colombia. Yet estimates of the total annual value added (profits) of the Colombian cocaine industry range from $2 billion to $10 billion (Economist, 2001b: 9; Lee, 1999:
33–34; Thoumi, 1999: 121). Leftist guerillas thus account for at most one-
quarter, and perhaps as little as 2–3 percent of Colombia's cocaine profits.
The remainder is controlled by 'traditional' DTOs and their associated para-
militaries. The relatively small share of drug profits controlled by guerilla
groups reflects their involvement in the less profitable cultivation and initial
processing stages. There is "no information that any FARC or ELN units
have established international transportation, wholesale distribution, or
drug money laundering networks (USDOJ 2000: 6)."

PLAN COLOMBIA

Former President Andres Pastrana launched Plan Colombia in 1999. It was
then and remains under current president Alvaro Uribe an ambitious effort
to legitimize the state, establish control over the countryside, and combat the
drug trade. In its preface, Pastrana noted that the country's history of civil
and political instability

> has been feed and aggravated by the enormous destabilizing effects of drug
> trafficking, which, with vast economic resources has constantly generated
> indiscriminate violence while undermining our values, on a scale compara-
> ble only to the era of Prohibition in the United States (Pastrana, 1999: 1).

Perhaps the (unintended?) irony of this statement was lost on drug war
hawks in the United States, who were eager to provide support for an effort
to wrest control of coca producing regions in southern Colombia from the
FARC. The United States has pledged dozens of helicopters and other war
material, as well as training and support for three elite counter-narcotics bat-
talions (Kotler, 2000). While the desperate Colombian government has wel-
comed military aid, Colombian civil society and foreign observers have
criticized the escalation of civil conflict (Economist, 2001b: 4).

Moreover, the guerilla movements targeted in Plan Colombia have relatively little control over the cocaine trade. Even if the FARC and ELN could
be eliminated, Colombia's major DTOs could continue operations relatively
unscathed. Comforting rhetoric aside, Plan Colombia offers little hope for

long-term counter-narcotics successes. A former U.S. military intelligence expert offers an alternative explanation for U.S. commitment to removing leftist insurgents from southern Colombia:

> The development of the Cusiana and Cupiagua oil fields, with an estimated 1.2 billion and 1.5 billion barrels respectively–the exploitation of which would establish Colombia as an OPEC caliber production country–is crucial to the country's economic recovery. The protection and early development of these fields is the bottom line for Colombia. Since the discovery of the oil reserves, the government has begun to establish security zones around those two locations. The problem at hand is how to project a positive security image in order to convince investors that it is safe to finance petroleum production infrastructure (Holden-Rhodes, 1997: 101–102).

These fields are located within the sphere of influence of the FARC and ELN. The rebels must be eliminated or suppressed for them to be developed (Holden-Rhodes, 1997: 103). In 2002, President Pastrana invited the U.S. to further expand its involvement in Colombia's civil conflict by providing security for oil infrastructure. He commented: "Today, the world is ready to unite against those who are attacking the interests of nations–and in this case the interest is energy (BBC News, 2002)." Military aid to Colombia seems more likely to enhance U.S. national oil security than it is to provide a viable solution to the cocaine problem.

Colombia's varied location specific advantages combine with significant early mover advantages to maintain the dominant position of Colombian DTOs. The cocaine trade flourishes in the violent disorder of Colombia's delegitimized state and fractured civil society. A glaring lack of comparable licit income options pushes peasants into the cultivation and initial processing of coca leaves. The refining, smuggling, and distribution stages have become more decentralized over time (both in space and in the number of market participants), making effective law enforcement more difficult.

The most serious challenge to Colombian traffickers has come not from the state, but from competitors. Mexican DTOs enjoy a number of distribution advantages and have steadily squeezed the Colombians out of profitable U.S. channels. In response, some Colombian groups have specialized in refining and smuggling, leaving U.S. distribution to Mexican, Dominican, or Jamaican DTOs. Others have aggressively exploited the growing European market, forming partnerships with 'local' enterprises (especially Russian mafias) to develop distribution networks. Both approaches have been successful, and the control of the cocaine industry by Colombian DTOs has not diminished appreciably.

Chapter Five
Cocaine Distribution and Mexico's Growing Competitive Advantage

Colombian firms have historically dominated the refining and smuggling of cocaine because they possessed the requisite connections, expertise, and assets to maintain competitive advantages over their South American partners/rivals. An important element of this advantage was the network of alliances they developed with local partners in the Caribbean, and (later) in Mexico and Central America. These relationships eased the trans-shipment of Colombian cocaine through the 'transit zone' and into the United States (Maingot, 1999).

Partnerships with Colombian traffickers stimulated the professional development of 'local' DTOs by providing them access to supplies of cocaine, weaponry, and other equipment. They also learned and adapted from their gained experience and 'knowledge spillovers' from Colombian firms. Emerging DTOs from a number of Caribbean countries (especially Jamaica, the Dominican Republic, Puerto Rico, and recently Haiti) have become more sophisticated and ambitious through these associations (USDOJ, 2000a). As transit zone DTOs matured, they eventually developed their own wholesale distribution networks in the U.S. This development changed the terms of their subcontracting relationships with Colombian producers, such that they could be simultaneously partners and competitors. Nowhere has this important shift been as evident as in Mexico, where local DTOs have grown rapidly in scale, power, and sophistication over the past 15 years. The development of the Mexican cocaine trade and its 'local' sources of competitive advantage are the primary focus of this chapter.

The value added to cocaine during the trans-shipment stage is considerable. A bulk shipment (tons) in Colombia is worth roughly $1200 per kilogram, but ten to twenty times that amount in wholesale markets of major

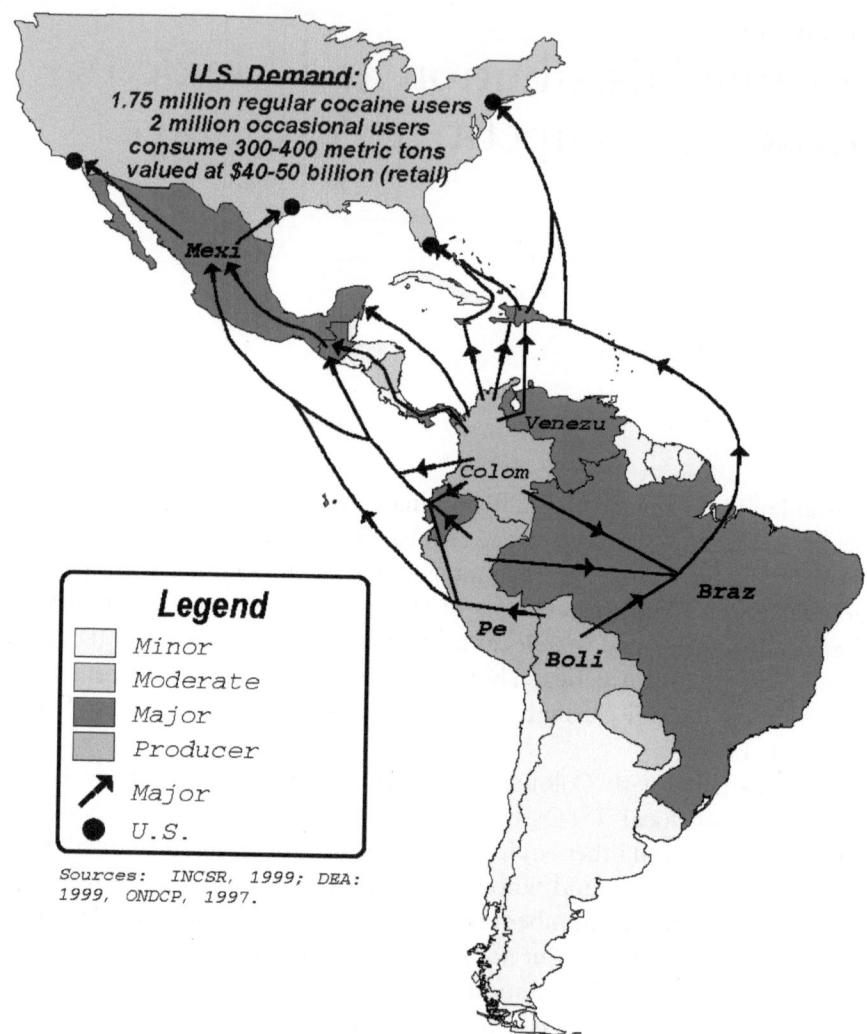

Figure 5.1 Major Cocaine Smuggling Routes

U.S. 'entry' cities. A portion of this added value reflects the risk of losing cargo and equipment during smuggling operations. Caulkins, et al. (1993) estimated that DTOs lose a third of shipments in the transit zone, either by interdiction or accident. Traffickers see these losses as a cost of doing business, and a portion of the value added is a risk premium reflecting these costs. Perhaps one fifth of transportation costs from source countries to the U.S. are accounted for by bribes to local officials in the transit zone (Maingot, 1999: 151).

The remainder of added value is accounted for by the transaction costs of exchanges between the various criminal actors involved in the trans-shipment process. Shipments may change hands several times along indirect smuggling routes from South America to the U.S. For example, the refiner might consign a load of cocaine to a shipper who moves it out of Colombia to Venezuela where another shipper takes over. It might then be shipped to Jamaica to further confuse interdiction efforts (Griffith, 1997: 89). Eventually a trafficker specializing in smuggling loads into the U.S. will deliver the shipment to a safe house.

Smugglers use a variety of transportation resources to move cocaine through the transit zone, including trucks, small commuter planes, commercial airliners, containerized cargo ships, and pleasure craft. Historically, air traffic has been the most favored method. Small commuter planes, laden with anywhere from 200 to 1,000 kg of cocaine delivered shipments from staging areas in Colombia to safe warehousing locations in Central America and the Caribbean (Riley, 1996: 209). Commercial airliners carrying multi-ton loads were occasionally used as well. Drug flights used a few major air corridors to take advantage of the region's minimal radar coverage and abundant private airstrips (Holden-Rhodes, 1997: 124).

In recent years, airborne shipments of cocaine have declined in favor of maritime smuggling, partly in response to the effectiveness of U.S. radar networks in closing off air routes to the U.S. (Holden-Rhodes, 1997: 125). Ships can also carry larger loads, making them more cost-effective. Smugglers may

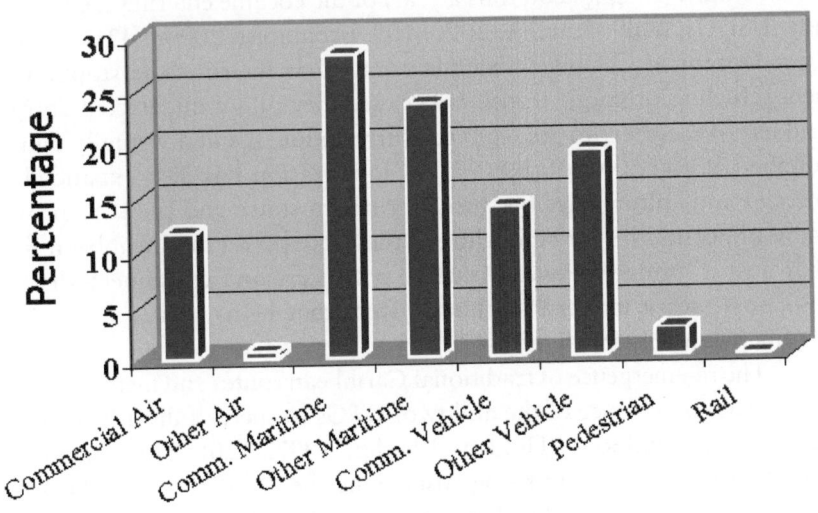

Figure 5.2 Border Cocaine Seizure by Smuggling Platform

use fishing vessels, pleasure craft, and 'go-fast' boats to move loads into the United States or to nearby staging locations like Mexico, Jamaica, Puerto Rico, the Dominican Republic, or Haiti (USDOJ, 2001c; USDOJ, 2000a). Detection of shipments hidden on container ships packed with legitimate cargo is even more challenging. Successful maritime interdiction is therefore reliant on detailed intelligence.

Figure 5.2 provides a general idea of what conveyances are used to smuggle cocaine into the U.S., but does not reflect the fact that seizure rates differ by smuggling method. For this reason, the prominence of some methods will be underestimated using seizure data. A good example is rail; the fact that no seizures have occurred in rail cars does not mean that rail assets are not being used. In fact, rail cars are an increasingly important method used along the U.S.—Mexico border.

THE CARIBBEAN ROUTE

The Caribbean has served as a major conduit for U.S. bound cocaine since the early years of the cocaine boom in the 1970s. A decade later, aggressive U.S. interdiction efforts in and around Florida stimulated traffickers to develop alternative routes. While never disappearing entirely, the Caribbean route faded in importance throughout much of the late 1980s and 1990s, while the 'Pacific' route through Mexico was favored. In recent years, Colombian DTOs have re-emphasized traditional Caribbean smuggling routes and the region is now used to transport most of the cocaine bound for Europe, and about a third (roughly 200 tons a year) of the cocaine entering the U.S. annually (USDOJ, 2000: 3; ICTA, 2000: 109; Economist, 2000d: 42).

Dozens of Caribbean islands are used as intermediate stops for storage, refueling or cargo transfers because they allow undetected entry into and use of their territories from the surrounding sea at a virtually unlimited number of places (Griffith, 1997). Globalization has also expanded commercial and cultural ties between Caribbean states and the U.S.–providing more opportunities for smuggling in the process. Yet the Caribbean is more than just a 'bridge' between cocaine producers and consumers–the region also possesses a modern banking system that helps shelter the industry's profits (Maingot, 1994: 470–472).

The re-emergence of traditional Caribbean routes and methods (e.g. 'go-fast' boats) is evidence of the ability of DTOs to successfully adapt to changing market conditions (Holden- Rhodes, 1997: 120). This ongoing shift results in large part from rising costs along the 'Pacific' route. The growing power of Mexican DTOs has enhanced their bargaining position with Colombian producers. The surcharge for moving shipments through Mexico

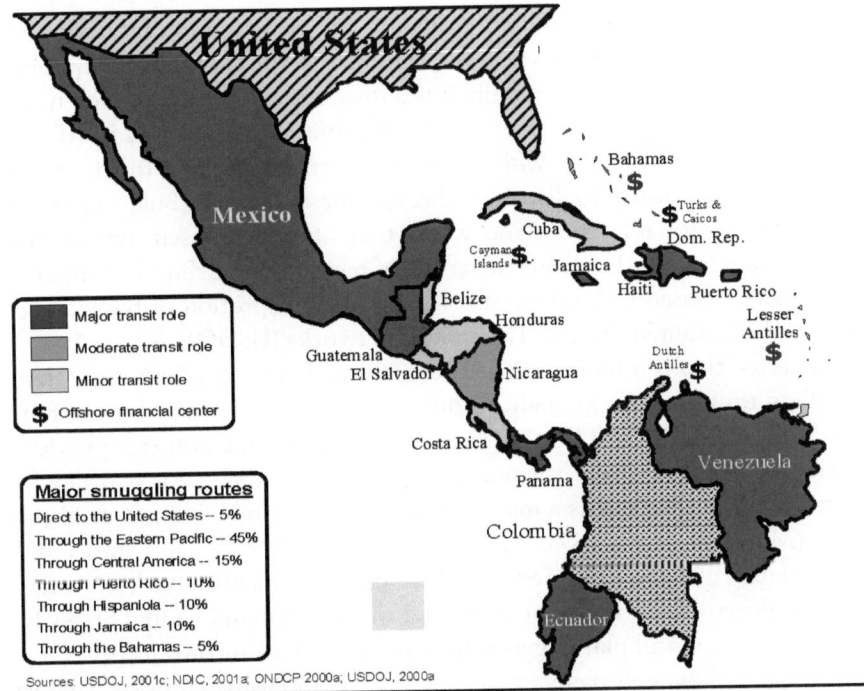

Figure 5.3 Cocaine Transit Zone

has risen to fifty percent of shipments, while Caribbean DTOs charge less than half that (Maingot, 1999: 146). Mexican DTOs have also developed reliable U.S. distribution networks and taken downstream market share away from Colombian groups. U.S. enforcement authorities argue that intensified inter-diction efforts at the Southwest border have also raised costs along the Pacific route (USDOJ, 2001: 1).

The primary South American staging area for the Caribbean route is Colombia's Guajira peninsula. The state has only a nominal presence in this sparsely populated region, isolated by the high peaks of the Santa Marta range (Riley, 1996: 209). Despite the Guajira Peninsula being less than 1,500 miles from the United States, direct shipments are uncommon because of radar detec-tion and the careful monitoring of U.S. coasts. The need for indirect routing to help conceal the source and nature of shipments has encouraged the develop-ment of satellite command and control centers by Colombian DTOs in the Dominican Republic, Puerto Rico and Haiti. Such commitments reflect both the critical role of these particular trans-shipment locations, as well as the need for Colombian managers to actively manage these relationships (USDOJ, 2000: 4).

The influence of Colombian DTOs on the growth and maturation of Caribbean criminal enterprises is most prominent in the Dominican Republic. Dominican groups have successfully established an extensive and well-managed wholesale distribution network throughout the Eastern U.S. (ICTA: 2000: 111). Deepening ties with Colombian groups provide them with a steady supply of cocaine to distribute through these channels. Bulk shipments are commonly flown to the island where they are warehoused, repackaged and smuggled into the U.S. using a variety of methods. The shipments are delivered to U.S.-based Colombian wholesalers, with a portion of the load retained and distributed through Dominican networks (USDOJ, 2001a: 1).

Puerto Rico is a major regional commercial port handling more than 14 million tons of cargo annually–figures that make it the third busiest port in the U.S. (ICTA, 2000: 111). This heavy volume of licit commerce provides a variety of opportunities for smuggling contraband–the major reason why Puerto Rico has emerged as a major entrepôt for Colombian and Caribbean DTOs (Maingot, 1999: 167). A second reason is Puerto Rico's status as a point of entry into the United States. Once drug shipments have been smuggled into Puerto Rico, they can be moved to the mainland United States by commercial ships and planes generally not subject to Customs inspections.

As U.S. law enforcement agencies have intensified efforts against smuggling through Puerto Rico and the Dominican Republic, Colombian DTOs have responded by routing more shipments through Jamaica and Haiti (Economist, 2002: 34; Rosenberg, 2000). Jamaica's long coastline, weak law enforcement, long-standing smuggling and distribution networks and close proximity to the U.S. make it a key staging area. Jamaican traffickers carefully manage the movement of cocaine through Jamaica into the U.S., and have developed in-house capacity for wholesale distribution and money laundering (Maingot, 1999: 158). Haiti is quickly developing into a major trans-shipment destination by exploiting its 'advantages'—weak democratic institutions, feeble law enforcement, poverty, and an accessible location along major Caribbean smuggling routes (Faul, 2000). This shift is only the most recent demonstration of operational flexibility by DTOs, which have developed alternative smuggling routes throughout the Caribbean and Eastern Pacific over the past two decades in response to interdiction efforts (McCaffery, 1999: 9).

Similar efforts to decentralize smuggling operations and dilute law enforcement attention involve Colombian DTOs and Venezuelan partners. Expanding trade ties between the two countries have increased the flow of Colombian cocaine through Venezuela's large, modern port facilities (Holden-Rhodes, 1997: 117). Colombian DTOs subcontract smuggling services to local enterprises, which transport shipments directly or indirectly to the U.S. hidden in commercial cargo (USDOJ, 2001c: 10). Menzel (1997: 169) estimates that the Cali 'cartel' moved more than 200 tons of cocaine through Venezuela annually. The country's relatively well-developed chemical and financial sectors make it an important source of precursor chemicals and a money-laundering center as well.

THE PACIFIC ROUTE

In 1988, approximately one-fifth of U.S. bound cocaine was smuggled through Mexico (Riley, 1996: 182). A decade later this figure had risen to approximately two-thirds of the total (NDIC, 2001; USDOJ: 1999: 9, USDOS, 1999: 1). Traffickers determined that the 'Pacific' route was not only a viable alternative, but was probably the optimal choice given the continued success of the U.S. radar barrier in the Caribbean (Economist, 1997a: 36).This shift in smuggling patterns is a clear example of the "balloon effect" first discussed in Chapter Two. The rise to prominence of Mexican DTOs represents a significant and unforeseen implication of U.S. efforts to disrupt drug flows through Florida and the Caribbean.

The first of two major sub-routes through the Pacific corridor uses aircraft, trucks, and maritime assets to move shipments through Central America. Roughly a quarter of the cocaine eventually smuggled into the U.S. from Mexico follows this route (USDOJ, 2001c: 2). Columbian DTOs maintain ownership of the shipments, but depend on local organization to

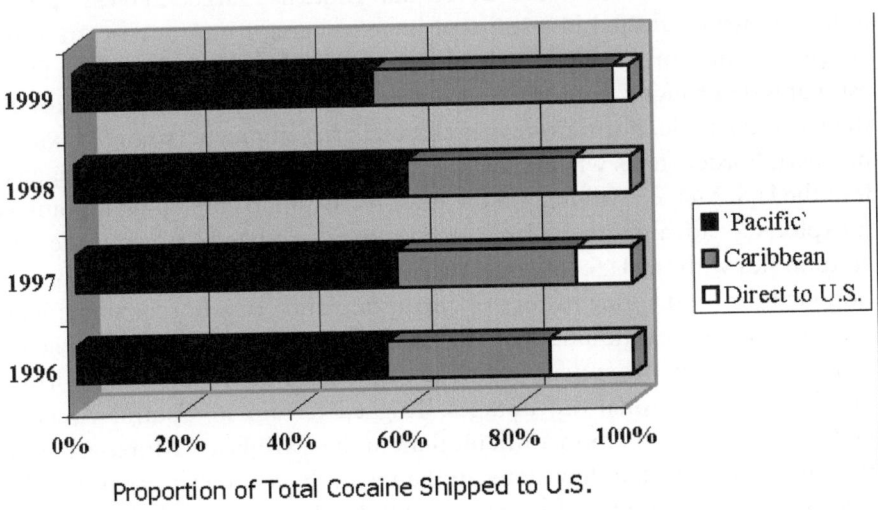

Figure 5.4 Relative Importance of Smuggling Routes

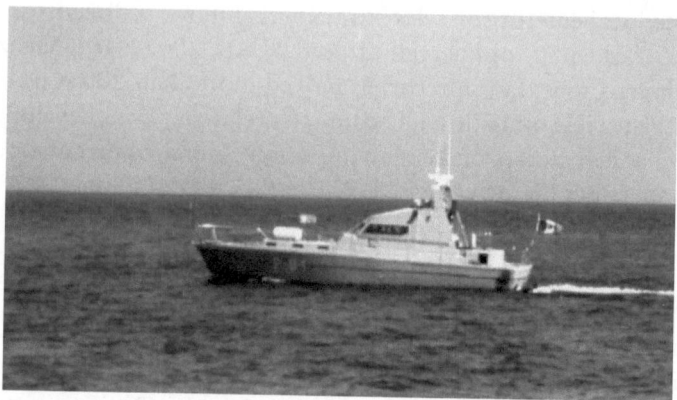

A Mexican naval vessel patrols the 300-mile Caribbean coastline of the state of Quintana Roo, long known as a major cocaine trafficking channel. Former Governor Mario Villanueva and his son were recently charged with narcotics conspiracy for accepting $45 million dollars from the Southeast 'Cartel' for protecting their shipments (USDOJ, 2002).

arrange transportation into Mexico (ICTA, 2000: 114). The second major sub-route transits the vast Eastern Pacific ocean using a variety of maritime assets, especially fishing vessels and 'go fast' boats. These shipments often originate in or around Buenaventura, the major port in Valle de Cauca department, historically a center of the Colombian cocaine business. Ecuadorian ports like Esmeraldas and Guayaquil are used as well (Holden-Rhodes, 1997: 126). Use of the 'EPAC' sub-route has surged in recent years, a development reflected in a series of huge (ranging from four to ten tons) cocaine seizures on fishing vessels in the region (USDOJ, 2001c). The DEA estimates that roughly half of all cocaine destined for the U.S. passes through the Eastern Pacific. Both sub-routes channel drug shipments to the Mexico's northern border states where they are warehoused and eventually smuggled into the U.S. Mexico will remain the most important transshipment point as it exploits its advantages: its long, porous northern border; deep trade and cultural ties with the U.S., relatively well developed port and air transportation facilities, and a long history of corruption and cross-border smuggling.

It is worth mentioning that DTOs in other countries along the Pacific route also occupy prominent positions in the cocaine trade by capitalizing on *their* own 'national' advantages. Rugged terrain in Central America makes radar detection more difficult than in the Caribbean. Moreover, even if flights were detected, few states in the region have aircraft capable of intercepting cocaine flights (Economist, 1997b). This fact symbolizes the region's general lack of capacity for responding to drug trafficking. More troubling are the region's weak political institutions, which are highly vulnerable to corruption.

After Mexico, the most entrepôt in the region is Guatemala, where Colombian DTOs operate a significant supply hub (Robinson, 1994: 449). After refining in Colombia, cocaine is transported here by plane to secure caches from which it can be easily moved into Mexico by land, sea or air (Holden-Rhodes, 1997: 156). The nearly 1,000 kilometer long border between Mexico and Guatemala is characterized by rough terrain, low population densities, and corrupt military and police institutions on both sides. The country has more than 2,000 legal or clandestine landing strips, which serve more than 100 drug flights a month (Holden-Rhodes, 1997: 134). Shipments are also occasionally transported directly to the U.S. hidden on container cargo ships.

Panama is a major commercial hub with large and modern trade and financial sectors. It has long been used by Colombian DTOs to smuggle shipments in commercial cargo and as a major money-laundering center. Modern seaports adjacent to the Colon Free Zone and at the Pacific end of

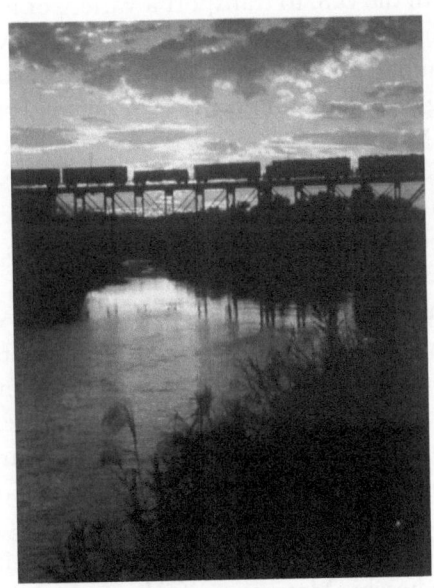

More trains cross the Mexican border at Laredo, TX than anywhere else. Growing rail traffic concerns law enforcement authorities, who suspect that an unknown but substantial amount of cocaine is concealed within them. The detection of drug shipments on trains is especially challenging and anti-narcotics efforts have had minimal success in countering this method.

the Panama Canal handle large volumes of containerized and bulk cargo and are important terminals for transshipping Colombian cocaine in and out of Panama (ICTA, 2000: 112). Honduras is another increasingly important link in the the Pacific route. Its long Atlantic coastline provides hundreds of deserted beaches perfect for drug trafficking. Another important advantage for traffickers is the country's lack of law enforcement capacity, notable even by Central American standards. The entire budget for all anti-narcotics operations in Honduras amounts to less than $1 million a year (Economist, 1997b: 50). The remainder of this chapter details Mexico's role in the international trans-shipment of cocaine, again illustrating how local conditions contribute to the development of competitive advantage in the cocaine trade.

CASE STUDY: MEXICO

Drug trafficking in Mexico is controlled by roughly 150 to 200 organizations, frequently comprised of close-knit family units (Holden-Rhodes, 1997: 85; Smith, 1999: 198). These groups are based primarily in the northern border states and take advantage of the region's deep cultural and economic linkages with the U.S. to transport a variety of illicit goods across the border. Many of these networks are generations old, having originated in the 1910s as gun running gangs during the Mexican Revolution. For the next decade, they smuggled alcohol into the U.S. during Prohibition. Beginning in the 1930s, the Mexican state pursued nationalist economic policies, attempting to restrict the importation of foreign goods. For four decades, smuggling clans earned huge profits smuggling consumer goods into Mexico from the U.S., circumventing Mexico's high tariff rates (Economist, 1997d: 37). As the Mexico government implemented market-oriented reforms in the 1980s, these organizations branched out into drug smuggling.

    In the early years of Colombian-Mexican partnerships, from the mid to late 1980s, traffickers in Mexico were essentially transportation sub-contractors. They moved Colombian cocaine through Mexico and across the U.S. border, where they delivered shipments to warehouses owned by Colombian distributors. For this service they were paid $1500–2000 per kilogram (USDOJ, 1999). The arrangement evolved as Mexican syndicates became more powerful. They renegotiated a payment-in-kind scheme with the Colombians, whereby Mexican traffickers would receive a portion of each shipment they moved across the border (Economist, 1997d: 37). It was cheaper for Colombian DTOs to turn over cocaine as payment for services, and Mexican organizations could make greater profits moving cocaine through their own distribution channels (Riley, 1996: 182).

Mexican traffickers could now exploit lucrative wholesale cocaine markets in the U.S. They quickly expanded their own distribution networks, a relatively simple task given the widespread and sizable population of Mexican origin in the U.S. By the early 1990s, roughly a dozen major Mexican DTOs and scores of minor ones waged increasingly violent turf wars against one another for control of this lucrative trade. Out of this competition rose the "Lord of the Skies" to prominence. Juarez-based Amado Carillo Fuentes began his trafficking career in the 1980s as a transportation subcontractor for Colombian producers. It was he who had changed the way business was conducted with the Colombians, receiving cocaine rather than cash (Economist, 1997d: 37).

He eventually implemented an innovative smuggling tactic by using jet airliners (hence the nickname) to transport multi-ton cocaine shipments into Mexico and the U.S (Holden-Rhodes, 1997: 143). By the mid 1990s, Mexican DTOs dominated cocaine distribution in the West and Midwestern U.S., while Colombians maintained their hold in the East (USDOJ, 1999). By 1997, however, rivals had diminished Carillo's base of power and the protection afforded him through his relationships with ranking police, military, and political authorities had faded. As law enforcement pressure mounted, Carillo underwent plastic surgery to change his appearance. He is thought to have died when surgeons mismanaged the administration of a drug used in the procedure—their gruesomely tortured corpses later turned up in barrels of concrete (Economist, 1997a).

The Tijuana-based Arellano Felix syndicate filled the power vacuum left by Carillo's apparent demise after a savage period of gang warfare (Smith, 1999). This clan is led by the nephews of imprisoned drug lord Miguel Angel Félix Gallardo, a former police officer who was among the first Mexican traffickers to establish relationships with Colombian DTOs in the mid 1980s (Padgett and Shannon, 2001). The Tijuana gang's extraordinary wealth, flamboyant leadership, and penchant for violence have earned it the distinction of being Mexico's most notorious and prominent drug trafficking organization (USDOJ, 2000: 45). While the group dominates the lucrative western-most section of the border by force, it does not hold monopoly power in drug trafficking.

A half-dozen other major Mexican DTOs operate out of their own bases in the border region (Smith, 1999: 198). These business-minded groups are no less successful, but maintain a lower profile. They comprise the top layer of the Mexican cocaine trafficking hierarchy. A middle tier is comprised of roughly a dozen smaller groups with fewer resources and modest distribution networks. These organizations can operate independently,

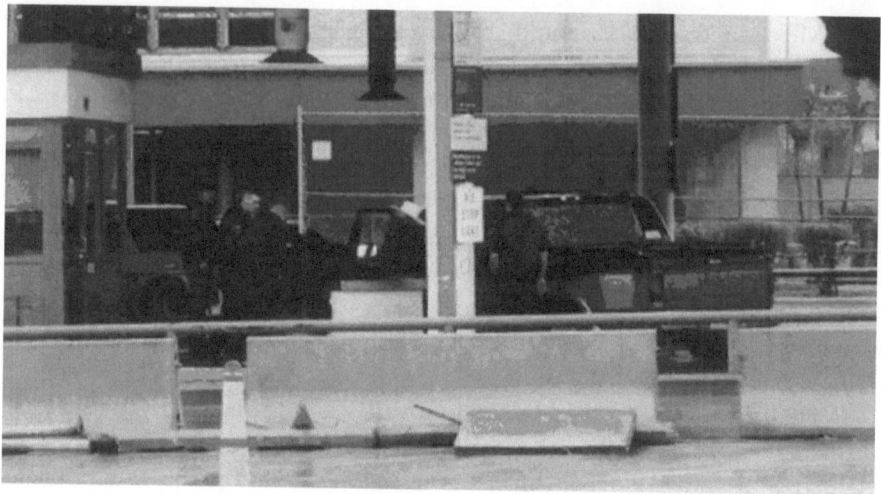

In December, 2000, DEA Operation Impunity II ended with the arrest of fifty members of a drug distribution enterprise based in Brownsville, TX. Cells of the organization were identified in McAllen, TX, Houston, Chicago, Columbus, Memphis and New York City. The operation became necessary when evidence emerged that the group had re-organized itself, with new distribution cell managers in the U.S. and management personnel in Mexico, after its apparent demise in Operation Impunity I (USDOJ, 2000c).

but often collaborate with the major trafficking groups in subsidiary roles. The bottom tier is comprised of scores of minor DTOs operating on both sides of the border. These provide specialized smuggling, warehousing, packing, transportation, and financial services for major Mexican and Colombian DTOs (USDOJ, 2001d). Due to the number of market participants, anti-drug operations against traffickers have minimal long-term effect on the cross-border drug trade. Remaining DTOs simply expand their own operations to include the routes or markets once served by dismantled organizations.

CORRUPTION

By the mid 1990s, drug trafficking played an undeniably important role in Mexico's economy. Estimates of the annual revenues of Mexico's drug traffickers run as high as $800 billion (Holden-Rhodes, 1997: 142). While this particular figure seems far-fetched, even conservative estimates of Mexican illicit drug revenues ($30–40 billion annually) suggest that the drug trade is Mexico's largest foreign exchange earner (Andreas, 1999a: 129). As the

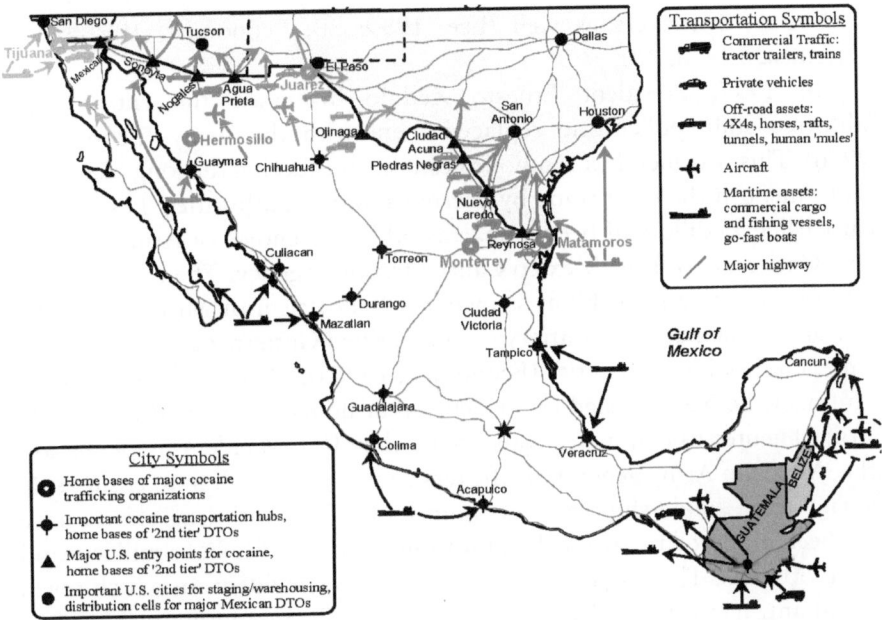

Figure 5.5 Cocaine Trafficking Through Mexico

trade flourished, power passed from small smuggling clans to larger, more sophisticated, business oriented organizations (Smith, 1999: 195). The need for capital and the rapid pace of privatization during the Salinas administration (1988–1994) had allowed drug lords to purchase banks and other enterprises with their fortunes. Seduced by huge bribes, high-ranking politicians, police officials, and military officers formed strong ties with the emerging drug mafia (Castañeda, 1995: 170). Over time, the distinction between drug lord, businessman, and politician became less evident. This official complicity was undoubtedly a significant factor in the rise and persistence of major Mexican DTOs (Schulz and Williams, 1995: 10).

Cases of high-level corruption in the police, military, and judiciary are so common that individual cases hardly merit mention. Mexican officials estimate that more than half of the Federal Judicial Police is on the payroll of one trafficking syndicate or another (Oppenheimer, 1996: 302). Corruption in state and local police forces is even more prevalent. The director of the U.S. Drug Enforcement Agency remarked, "there is not one single law-enforcement institution in Mexico with which the DEA has an entirely trusting relationship (Economist, 1997c: 26)." U.S. federal authorities admit that police officials and judges on the U.S. side of the border are on the payroll of Mexican traffickers as well (Lee, 1999: 30; Economist, 1997c: 25; Economist, 1997d: 38).

In 1997, President Ernesto Zedillo dismissed the entire Baja California state police and replaced them with the Army (Economist, 1997d). This was merely a symbolic gesture, considering the long history of involvement in the drug trade by corrupt military authorities. Less than a year earlier, Zedillo had been embarrassed by his choice of Army General Jesus Gutierrez to head Mexico's anti-narcotics agency. The appointment had been an attempt to blunt stringent U.S. criticism of Mexican efforts. U.S. 'drug czar' Barry McCaffery even described Gutierrez as "a guy of absolute, unquestioned integrity (Economist, 1997a)." Yet weeks after his appointment, he was arrested on evidence that he had been paid by Amado Carillo Fuentes to eliminate rivals. In another 1997 incident involving another Mexican Army general, traffickers provided $1 million to ensure safe passage for a single shipment (Economist, 1997c). Anti-drug efforts have long been hindered by strained relationships between Mexican military and police officials. These date to an infamous 1991 incident, in which seven federal anti-narcotics policemen were killed while attempting to capture a cocaine-laden plane. The gunmen were part of a local army unit that had been contracted to protect traffickers as they refueled U.S. bound drug flights (Oppenheimer, 1996: 301).

These incidents are only the most visible examples of the inexorable linkages between law enforcement officials and narco-traffickers in Mexico. While the depth and breadth of corruption hinted at by these events is shocking, the enormous amount of money available to DTOs for bribing officials at least makes it understandable. Tijuana's Arellano brothers alone spend $50–75 million annually on payoffs to local, state and federal officials (Padgett and Shannon, 2001; Economist, 1997d: 38). The total spent on bribery by all Mexican traffickers is perhaps $500 million a year (Smith 1999: 204).

The most notable case of high-level corruption involved former President Salinas' brother and right-hand man, Raúl. Persuasive allegations link Raúl Salinas to prominent drug trafficker Juan Garcia Abrego, head of the powerful Gulf 'cartel' (Anderson, 1996). With Salinas in a position of power, Abrego could act with impunity, as local officials understood that he had protection at the highest levels (Economist, 1997d). After his brother Carlos left office in 1994, Raúl was arrested and convicted of illegal enrichment. Abrego was then arrested and extradited to the U.S., where he is currently serving life in prison. Raúl's involvement in the drug-related 1994

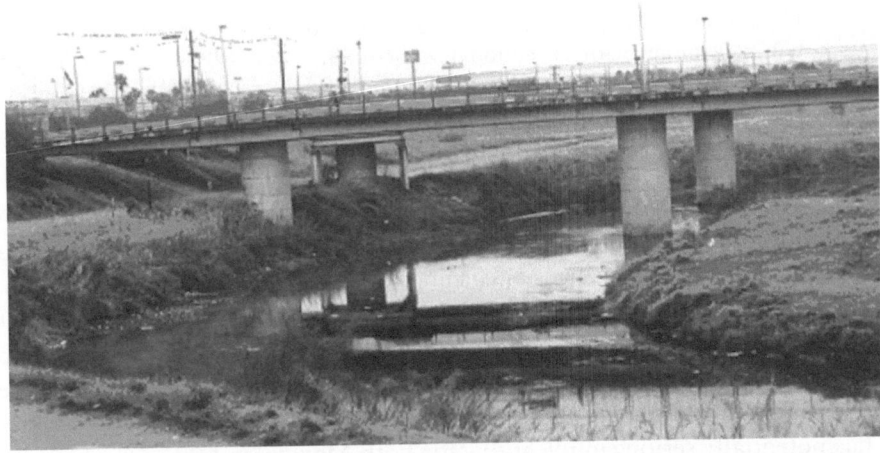

Bridge connecting Brownsville, TX with Matamoros, Mexico. Juan Garcia Abrego's once-dominant Gulf 'cartel' was based here. After his 1996 imprisonment, cocaine trafficking in northeast Mexico became more decentralized. Numerous smaller, specialized DTOs currently operating there have made South Texas the border's most prominent smuggling region.

murder of prominent ruling party politician José Francisco Ruiz Massieu also raised questions about the nature of the Salinas family's ties to drug trafficking (Smith, 1999: 203; Gray, 1998: 140; Schulz and Williams, 1995: 19–25). Carlos Salinas has denied involvement from Ireland, where he has resided since his presidential term ended.

It seems possible that President Salinas might have forged some sort of agreement with Mexico's drug bosses during his term. His primary goal would have been to encourage them to invest their earnings in Mexico, thus helping to ease the country's debt problem. It was also desirable that traffickers employ greater discretion to avoid embarrassing the Mexican government or drawing the attention of U.S. authorities. Such concerns were critically important to the Salinas administration, especially during the negotiation and ratification of the North American Free Trade Agreement (NAFTA). In return for meeting these two goals, traffickers would be allowed to proceed with their activities with minimal state interference (Castaneda, 1995: 167).

The emergence and persistence of exceptionally powerful and well-connected drug trafficking organizations raises concerns about the potential 'Colombianization' of Mexican politics and society (Holden-Rhodes, 1997: 136). Smith (1999: 203) notes:

Expansion of the Mexican drug trade caught the nation's political system at a moment of exceptional vulnerability. The 1990s have been marked by disintegration, liberalization, incipient reconstruction—and pervasive uncertainty. In the short run, the process of "democratization" in Mexico has probably eased working conditions for the traficantes.

Yet there are important differences in the social, political, and economic characteristics of the two countries. The cocaine trade is relatively less important in Mexico in terms of earnings or employment. While corruption, political unrest, and crime are certainly problems in Mexico, they are not yet at the same scale or scope as in Colombia. Mexico's political system also seems more transparent and its civil society more vibrant. Nonetheless, the introduction of drug profits into Mexico's legitimate economy and politics has potentially serious implications for both Mexico and the U.S.

ECONOMIC INTEGRATION

Two broad processes account for the expansion of cocaine trafficking activities in Mexico. The first was the intensification of U.S. anti-narcotics efforts targeting Florida and the Caribbean in the mid 1980s. These operations raised risks and costs along the region's deeply entrenched smuggling routes. Colombian DTOs quickly moved to develop partnerships with Mexican criminal groups to secure alternative routes through Mexico. This expansion of Mexico's role in the cocaine trade was greatly facilitated by a concurrent and sweeping program of market oriented economic reform that intensified during the presidency of Carlos Salinas (1988–1994). These reforms were intended to help Mexican enterprises to take advantage of the country's comparative advantages and become internationally competitive exporters. Unfortunately, Mexican drug trafficking syndicates were and continue to be among the few domestic firms to realize this goal.

The success of Mexican DTOs reflects their ability to exploit Mexico's competitive advantages in drug trafficking. These include endemic corruption and widespread poverty, a long and vulnerable border with the U.S., extensive experience with cross-border smuggling, large migrant populations in the U.S., and strong and diverse economic linkages with the United States. The ability of Mexican traffickers to internalize and exploit such advantages has been enhanced by the program of privatization, trade liberalization, and deregulation implemented over the past fifteen years. Such efforts encourage both licit and illicit cross-border activities alike. Andreas (1999a) notes that market based reforms increase incentives to enter illicit industries, make it easier to launder profits, and generally hinder law enforcement efforts. A brief review of recent political economy in Mexico illustrates those aspects of the reform program most relevant to the cocaine trade.

By 1982, weakening oil markets made Mexico's $80 billion foreign debt an increasingly serious problem. Petroleum accounted for nearly three-quarters of Mexico's export earnings, and budget forecasts were based largely on increased oil prices and normal production levels (Krooth, 1995: 314). The worldwide oil glut meant actual revenues were far below projected levels. As foreign exchange earnings declined, Mexico's access to credit was reduced to the point where it defaulted on its foreign debt obligations. The immediate consequences were a dramatic decline in economic activity, and a significant increase in both unemployment and inflation (Teichman, 1995: 69).

Despite a series of adjustment programs and debt restructurings, Mexico soon exhausted both oil revenues and foreign debt as ways to subsidize protected domestic industries. The United States and international lending agencies pressured Mexico to adopt a program of market-based economic reform. These sought to expand Mexico's export potential by opening the economy to foreign trade, attracting foreign investment, cultivating the private sector, privatizing state industries, and cutting government spending (Otero, 1996: 7; LaBotz, 1995: 101–103). Such measures were a clear departure from the nationalist development policies Mexico had followed for the previous half century (Erfani, 1995: 163). The most important element of this reform program was the implementation of the NAFTA in 1994. The pact was the capstone of Salinas' renovation of the Mexican economy and sought to further liberalize cross-border trade and investment by eliminating remaining barriers to economic interaction (Schulz and Williams, 1995: 15). In this regard, it has been an unquestioned success.

Expanded trade flows between the U.S. and Mexico provide a wide variety of opportunities to conceal drugs within licit commercial traffic. Mexican DTOs have developed a number of sophisticated methods for doing so (ONDCP, 2000: 2). DEA officials concede that the majority of cocaine arrives through legal ports of entry, and have even characterized NAFTA as a "godsend" to large volume drug trafficking (Andreas, 1999: 134). Indeed, the workload of anti-narcotics agencies has increased dramatically as cross-border economic interaction has expanded. In 2000, 193 million people, 89 million cars, 4.5 million tractor-trailers, and 572,583 rail cars crossed into the U.S. from Mexico (U.S. Customs, 2000). A substantial portion of this traffic flows through Texas, with a notable concentration of activity along a two hundred mile stretch of border from Laredo to Brownsville. In this relatively densely settled region, communities and cultures on each side of the border are especially closely integrated.

Table 5.1 Total Mexican Imports and Exports to/from the United States

Year	Imports ($Billion)	% U.S. Total	Exports ($Billion)	% U.S. Total
1991	33.3	7.8%	31.1	6.4%
1992	40.6	9.1%	35.2	6.6 %
1993	41.6	8.9%	39.9	6.9 %
1994	50.8	9.8%	49.5	7.5 %
1995	46.3	7.9%	62.1	8.4 %
1996	56.8	9.1 %	74.3	9.3 %
1997	71.4	10.4%	85.9	9.9 %
1998	78.8	11.5%	94.6	10.4 %
1999	86.9	12.5%	109.7	10.7 %

Source: United States International Trade Administration, 1991–1999.

Interaction and integration in the U.S.-Mexico border region are so extensive that the region is increasingly recognized as a 'borderline nation,' distinct from both countries (Allen and deSocio, 2002). The environment provides limitless opportunities for drug smuggling, a fact recognized in official documents which note, "contributing to enforcement problems are border communities in the U.S. that are linked by common cultural, familial, commercial, and industrial ties or interests to neighboring Mexico (ONDCP, 2000: 2)." The South West Border Control Strategy developed by U.S. anti-narcotics authorities stresses the importance of the region to drug interdiction efforts and urges an expansion of the military's role in border defense (Holden-Rhodes, 1997: 86). This strategy fails, however, to address the obvious paradox between trade liberalization and drug prohibition. Andreas (1998: 203) observes:

> As old barriers between the United States and Mexico are being torn down under NAFTA and the two nations are drawn closer together, new barriers are rapidly being built up to keep them apart.

Since 1993, U.S. federal resources dedicated to drug-control along the Southwest border have increased dramatically. They now involve seven federal departments, more than 11,000 officials, and cost roughly $2 billion a year (McCaffery, 1998b). Nonetheless, the sheer extensiveness of the border region and the heavy volume of commercial traffic that cross at certain locations provide traffickers a variety of smuggling opportunities. A far more

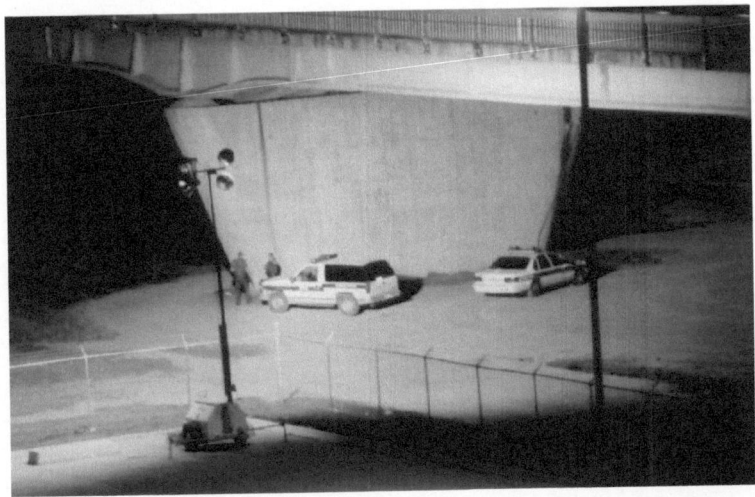

The Border Patrol maintains a highly visible presence throughout the border region. While their primary mission is to deter and intercept undocumented migrants, they play a major role in drug interdiction along the Southwest border.

intensive and intrusive inspection regime would be required to keep traffickers from using licit commercial means to smuggle shipments. The problem with intensified inspection programs is that they hinder legal commerce. This dilemma reflects a precarious balance of policies between drug enforcement and the facilitation of licit trade, that given current priorities and historical trends, will likely tip in favor of commerce. As Holden-Rhodes (1997: 166) notes, it is quite clear that political considerations . . . will ensure that trafficking issues will be checkmated by trade priorities." The implications of this decision for anti-narcotics efforts are obvious.

In light of these conditions, it seems likely that Mexican DTOs will continue to play a critical role in the delivery and distribution of cocaine within the United States. The continued development of economic, cultural and political linkages between the two countries has the unintended effect of enhancing the competitive advantages of Mexican traffickers. Yet closer relations with Mexico do fulfill a number of important U.S. economic and foreign policy objectives. To deny these in an attempt to curb drug trafficking would be a mistake.

Chapter Six

Marketing Cocaine in the United States

Cocaine shipments are smuggled into the United States at many locations, using an assortment of methods, and vary widely in size from a few kilograms to multi-ton lots. Once they enter the country, shipments are commonly consolidated in warehousing facilities near the point of entry. In these distribution hubs, loads are re-organized, re-packaged and stored in preparation for movement to downstream markets. Major drug trafficking organizations locate command and control 'cells' in these distribution centers. Regional managers supervise wholesale distribution networks and communicate directly with top-level management headquartered in home countries regarding the correct size, destination, and method of exchange for shipments (USDOJ, 2001c; USDOJ, 2000a: 3).

These are commonly ton-scale shipments meant to fill orders in a major market, and are commonly hidden within tractor-trailer shipments of legitimate cargo. Once loads are delivered to major wholesale connections in destination markets, they are distributed to street-level retail dealers through a multi-layered, hierarchical network of wholesale dealers. Caulkins (1997: 138–9) estimates that there are roughly a half million dealers involved with distributing cocaine in the United States. Most are concentrated at the retail end of the distribution process, and are not associated with multinational drug trafficking organizations.

The wholesale distribution of cocaine in the U.S. is functionally organized through a cell-based network. Cells operate within specific geographic areas and offer specialized transportation, storage, brokerage, or money laundering services (USDOJ, 2000: 36). To prevent the network from being infiltrated by counter-drug operations, operatives have little knowledge regarding the operations of other cells. Regional managers 'work' the U.S. network and communicate with supervisors in home countries. Cell members are occasionally rotated home to reinvigorate family and business connections, a practice also meant to confuse and counter law enforcement efforts (Filippone, 1994: 334).

A second method commonly used by DTOs to provide operational security is to develop, exploit, and then disband wholesale distribution cells in a continuous cycle. For example, a Mexican DTO will send agents to rent a safe house in a working-class neighborhood of a target market. Drugs are delivered in batches by affiliated transportation cells to the stash house from warehouses near the point of entry. Distribution cell members receive detailed instructions from managers in Mexico regarding amounts, prices, and delivery methods for numerous downstream wholesale exchanges. Transactions at this level are difficult targets for law enforcement because wholesalers are careful to sell only to 'screened' buyers. Customers are commonly Mexican nationals at least two levels removed from the retail market. After a few successful operations, the cell disbands and returns to Mexico (NDIC, 2001b: 8).

Mexican DTOs dominate wholesale cocaine distribution in the West and Midwestern United States and have steadily gained market share in the East, particularly in New York and Philadelphia (USDOJ, 2001c: 3). As Mexican groups expand eastwards, historically dominant Colombian traffickers have ceded distribution responsibilities to other organizations. Dominican, Jamaican or Haitian organizations now manage extensive distribution networks in the East (NDIC, 2001a). 'Ethnic' DTOs capitalize on the presence of affiliated migrant populations in developing distribution networks. Such strategies are important to minimizing the organization's risk exposure.

CENTRAL PLACE THEORY

The wholesale distribution of cocaine is modeled here using central place theory. This is a set of location principles that formalize the complex relationships regarding the size, spacing, distribution and service characteristics of cities in an urban hierarchy (Wheeler, et.al., 1998: 153). Settlements are termed central places because they are at the geographic and functional (market) center of an associated trade area. Large central places offer the greatest variety of goods and services. Residents of smaller settlements depend on larger central places for goods and services not available locally (Kolars and Nystuen, 1974: 78). The frictional effect of distance and presence of intervening opportunities determine the specific nature and location of this interaction.

All marketing activities can be ranked by the size of their threshold market, which represents the minimum demand necessary to sustain that activity (Jones and Simmons, 1990: 154). Goods or services with small threshold markets are considered low-order; those with large thresholds are high-order. Low-order goods are purchased more frequently and have smaller trade areas. They are sold in many locations with sellers relatively close to one another. Higher order goods are purchased less frequently, have larger trade areas, and are available from a smaller number of places (Hanink, 1997: 284). The cocaine trade encompasses a spectrum of marketing activities, each with a distinctive threshold market. Therefore, cocaine distribution activities can be ranked from low-order (street level, by-dose crack sales) to high-order (ton level wholesale transactions) activities.

The 'centrality' of any particular city in the urban hierarchy is measured by the highest-order good offered there. High-order goods are found only in high-order centers, whose trade areas contain the trade areas of numerous lower-order centers. Each higher level of the urban hierarchy offers a greater variety of goods and services from a smaller number of central places. In this manner, the ordering of goods and services by threshold size generates a hierarchy of nested spatial markets "optimally efficient in both demand and supply (Esparza and Krmenec, 1996: 368)." In this system,

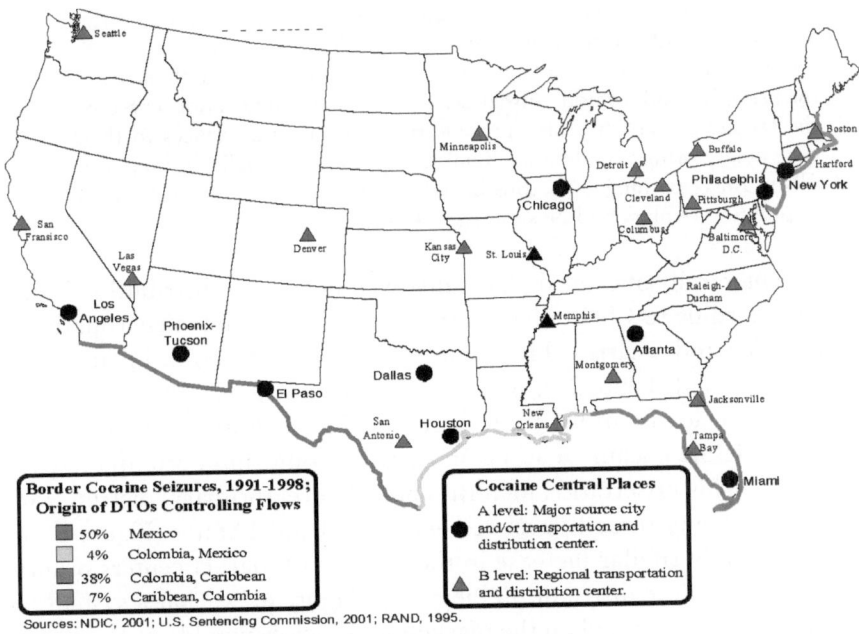

Figure 6.1 Cocaine Distribution Hierarchy of U.S. Cities

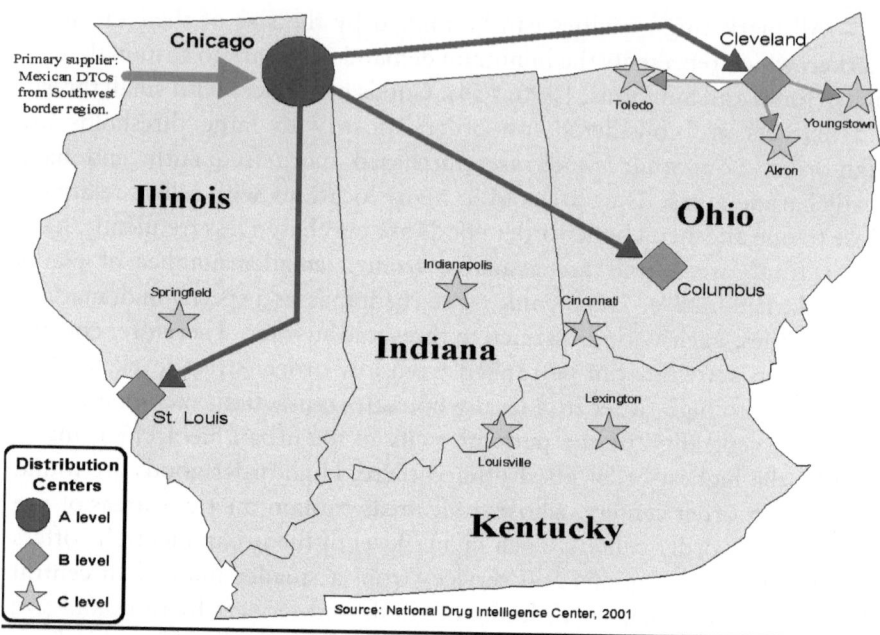

Figure 6.2 Cocaine Distribution in the Midwestern U.S.

a few large settlements furnish all customers with specialized services and also provide populations immediately adjacent to themselves with middle range services and basic necessities. Medium size settlements in turn supply similar middle-range services to all customers not served by the largest center; they also provide basic goods and services to their own neighboring populations. Finally, a network of small central places fills in the remaining gaps, thus bringing basic services to the rest of the population (Kolars and Nystuen, 1974: 80).

The hierarchy of central places involved in cocaine distribution is organized according to Christaller's marketing principle, in which a spatially dispersed demand is satisfied by a minimum number of central places (see Dicken and Lloyd, 1990: 28). In this system, each higher-order trade area contains three lower order trade areas ($k=3$, see Jones and Simmons, 1990). Wholesale cocaine markets in the U.S. conform approximately to this pattern. This dissertation identifies nine A-level (primary) distribution centers and twenty-three B-level centers in the United States (Figure 6.1). A proportionally similar increase in the number of market centers occurs at lower levels of the distribution hierarchy (Figure 6.2). That a system of cocaine distribution based on the marketing principle would emerge is not surprising. This type of hierarchy minimizes the number of transactions required to satisfy a spatially distributed demand. It therefore minimizes risk and transaction costs, both critical considerations in illicit commerce.

The cocaine distribution system is not, however, a strictly regimented and rational hierarchy. It does not conform perfectly to the geometry of the marketing principle, and centers do not serve exclusive market areas. While distribution centers do serve specific spatial markets, there are significant overlaps in trade areas. Such overlaps are, in fact, a common feature in many empirical applications of central place theory (Wheeler, et.al., 1998: 164). Few empirical studies that have identified a precise geometric pattern of nested markets as originally theorized in Christaller's pioneering work on central places (Esparza and Krmenec, 1996: 367). The geometric logic of any particular system of central places reflects a variety of influences; the density of settlements, obstacles to spatial interaction, transportation infrastructure, or the administrative history of the region (Krmenec and Esparza, 1999: 267; Dicken and Lloyd, 1990: 36; Jones and Simmons, 1990: 157). Real world city systems commonly display a mixture of Christaller's organizing principles, and often assume non-integral k values (Mulligan, 1984: 11). Changes in the nesting factors (k-values) have even been observed from one level of the hierarchy to the next within the same industry. Central place theory offers a flexible approach to the study of spatial systems, and is quite useful for explaining cocaine distribution despite the noted departures from idealized theoretical constructs.

At the top of the cocaine distribution hierarchy in the United States are nine A-level distribution centers, including five dual-role transportation hubs (NDIC, 2001a: 10). These five 'source cities' serve as the primary U.S. destinations for drug shipments and supply one or more other major distribution centers with bulk shipments. They also serve as A-level distribution centers, providing a wide range of distribution services to a regional trade area. Mexican DTOs operate transportation hubs in Los Angeles, Phoenix-Tucson, El Paso, and Houston (also used by Colombian DTOs). Miami is the final transportation hub, used by both Colombian and Caribbean-based DTOs. The other four A-level distribution centers are Atlanta, Chicago, New York City, and Philadelphia. These are major market centers supplied by one or more transportation hubs, which in turn supply cocaine to lower-order market centers in their region.

Distribution channels reflect the influence of both hierarchical and expansion diffusion processes. A ton-sized cocaine shipment might originate in Reynosa, Mexico and be smuggled across the border by a specialized cell to McAllen, TX. It would then be transported and warehoused in Houston, an

A-level distribution hub supplying multi-hundred kg lots to other A-level centers like Atlanta, Chicago, and New York. Distributors in Houston also have direct connections to regional B-level centers like New Orleans, Memphis, Montgomery, and Tampa Bay. 'Local' C level centers like Shreveport or Baton Rouge would also be supplied directly from Houston.

The preceding example indicates that the distribution process can 'skip' levels in the hierarchy, another departure from theoretical expectations of such systems. Caulkins (1995: 44) observes that cocaine is commonly shipped to lower-order distribution centers from a complex network of geographically dispersed origins. For example, Columbus, Ohio is a B-level center which is supplied not only from Chicago, the nearest A-level center, but also directly (to a lesser degree) from other A-level centers like Miami and New York City, as well as Detroit, a B-level center (NDIC, 2001a: 9). These 'redundant' supply connections reflect the presence of marketing cells from multiple DTOs, each with their local contacts and distribution channels. For example, Columbus is supplied by Mexican DTOs through Chicago and by Dominican groups through New York City (NDIC, 2001d: 2). C-level centers might be served from multiple A or B-level centers; for example, Cincinnati is supplied from both Chicago and Columbus.

Nonetheless, there is a clear hierarchy of distribution functions reflecting the ordering of centers. A-level centers have large multi-state trade areas and display a full range of distribution activities from retail sales to ton-level wholesale exchanges. B-level centers serve medium-sized regional trade areas and have a more limited range of distribution activities, including wholesale deals potentially involving tens or hundreds of kilograms. C-level centers serve smaller local trade areas, and have limited involvement in the bulk wholesale trade. Here, multi-kilogram transactions are the highest-order distribution function, with the largest common transaction involving multi-ounce lots. Lower-order centers serve smaller urban areas and provide only retail distribution functions. The largest transactions in a D-level center, for instance, would involve multi-gram lots, with exchanges of gram or smaller quantities most common.

The value of hierarchical diffusion processes for explaining the wholesale distribution of cocaine has been identified, but not fully developed, by other authors. Rengert (1996: 20) describes a system in which

> Drug distributors originate in the largest cities at the top of the country's hierarchy of central places and subsequently filter down in an orderly progression to metropolitan centers of decreasing size (Rengert, 1996: 20).

Caulkins (1995: 51) also identifies a hierarchical distribution pattern for cocaine among cities in the Mid-Atlantic—Great Lakes region. He observes significant differences in cocaine prices among what he called Tier I cities, Tier II cities and smaller cities. The existence of higher per unit prices in smaller markets is consistent with the notion that cocaine is distributed through an urban hierarchy where prices increase perceptibly with each step along the distribution chain.

COCAINE PRICE, PURITY AND MARKET SIZE

The relative importance, or centrality, of settlements in the cocaine distribution process provides insight regarding differences in cocaine prices from place to place. Low-order distribution centers are characterized by relatively high per-unit prices, while higher-order places have lower per-unit prices. Caulkins (1995: 40) observes:

> Prices are lower in larger and denser markets because of external economies of scale associated with the distribution of illicit drugs. Sources of these economies include diluting law enforcement pressure, reducing search times, and creating competitive pressures that make it difficult to extort monopoly rents.

External economies are indeed important, but do not fully account for price differences (NDIC 2001a: 2). The remainder is explained by distance and transportation costs, which increase directly with distance (geographical or hierarchical) from distribution central places. Freight rates, in a traditional sense, are relatively unimportant for cocaine, given its high value per unit weight. Variations in price indicate, instead, that the distribution process is characterized by significant transaction costs (Caulkins, 1995: 52). High unit prices in smaller markets reflect the actual and potential costs incurred by participants exposed to the risks and uncertainties of illicit market transactions. While significant transaction costs exist at all levels of the distribution hierarchy, they are incurred more often and spread among smaller volumes at downstream stages.

These factors generate a significant quantity discount for cocaine, with per unit prices varying dramatically between different levels of the distribution hierarchy. While quantity discounts exist for many licit products, they are more pronounced for cocaine due to the higher risks and transaction costs associated with illicit distribution (Caulkins, 1994: 815). Large quantity discounts make meaningful price comparisons between markets difficult, unless the transactions in question are of the same size and at the same level of the distribution hierarchy. Table 6.2 demonstrates the extent of

Table 6.1 Spatial and Scalar Differences in U.S. Cocaine HCl Prices

	Gram	Ounce	Kilogram
Atlanta	$100	$1,000	$23,000
Boston	$50–90	$650–1,400	$24,000–32,000
Chicago	$50–100	$1,000	$18,000–20,000
Denver	$80	$800–1,200	$18,000–22,000
Minneapolis	$100	$700–1,200	$24,000
New Orleans	$80–150	$800–1,200	$20,000–28,000
Phoenix	$80	$400–800	$13,500–17,000
Washington, D.C.	$100–200	$1050–1,200	$22,000–25,000
Texas	$50–125	$500–1,200	$10,000–22,000
New York City	$20–50	$650–1000	$20,000–28,000

Source: National Institute on Drug Abuse, 2000.

quantity discounts in cocaine markets. In Atlanta, for example, gram level transactions are more than 400% more expensive per unit weight than kilogram level exchanges. Significant differences in prices from city to city are not apparent in Table 6.2, probably because each of the cities included are major (A or B level) distribution centers.

It must be noted that these prices are not standardized to account for variations in purity. For price comparisons between one place and another to be meaningful, one must account for the purity of the cocaine exchanged, which decreases as it moves downstream to retail markets. At the bulk wholesale level, shipments of 80–90% purity are the norm (NDIC, 2001a: 2). In bulk retail markets, ounce quantities commonly range from 50–80% purity (USDOJ, 2001d). In one compilation of gram-level seizure data from across the country, purity levels ranged from 15–90% (ONDCP, 2001). Purity levels at this stage were found to be highest (roughly 80%) in A-level distribution centers like New York, Philadelphia, Miami, and Los Angeles. Average purity levels were significantly less (roughly 50%) in B-level centers like Denver, Seattle, and Memphis. Similar declines in purity likely occur at subsequently lower levels of the distribution hierarchy. Purity levels of seized cocaine may therefore offer greater insight regarding the distribution hierarchy than price data.

While drug related data is available from a number of law enforcement agencies, its collection is conducted haphazardly, with little or no concern given to representative sampling or standardization of methods or presentation. Price data is presented out of context and removed from the critical

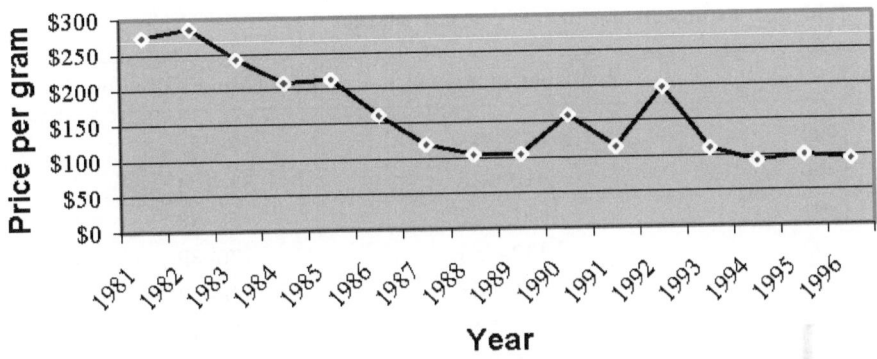

Figure 6.3 Wholesale Unit Prices of Cocaine HCl

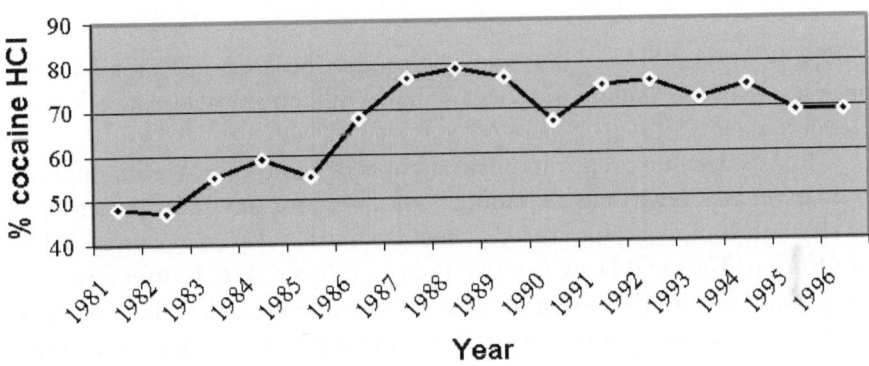

Figure 6.4 Wholesale Purity of Cocaine

considerations of either purity or lot size. Further confusion about prices is generated by the purposeful misrepresentation of the value of drug seizures by law enforcement agencies. Rengert (1996: 8) observes:

> the actual value of confiscated drugs may be relatively small when calculated back to the producing country rather than forwarding to street prices, as is the common law enforcement practice . . . confiscated drugs can be replaced easily at relatively low cost within producing nations.

While this is indeed true, neither forward nor backward calculations are appropriate methods for valuing seizures. Rather, a 'true' replacement value must be calculated at the stage in which the shipment was lost or seized. For example, a five hundred kilogram wholesale transaction seized in Houston is worth roughly $7.5 million (at $15,000 per kilogram), the cost to replace the shipment at that stage. The replacement costs are certainly more than

Table 6.2 Estimated Size of U.S. Cocaine Market

	Available Supply (Mt)	Retail Value ($ Billion)
1989	432–545	70–89
1990	413–528	82–104
1991	412–532	68–88
1992	437–555	70–89
1993	364–463	56–72
1994	258–345	36–48
1995	287–376	40–52

Source: Rhodes (ONDCP), 1997.

$600,000 (at $1,200 per kilogram), the production costs in Colombia, and much less than $45 million (the value of half a million gram dose units sold at a retail price of $90).

Just as cocaine price and purity figures demand critical examination, so do estimates regarding the number of users, consumption patterns, or the size and composition of the U.S. cocaine market. Estimates provided by the Office of National Drug Control Policy (Tables 6.3; 6.4) offer a reasonable general idea of the extent of cocaine use but have little value for measuring or predicting changes in demand or supply of cocaine over time, especially over short periods. Close examination of the figures raises immediate questions that reinforce the importance of viewing drug related data with healthy suspicion.

Table 6.3 Cocaine Consumption Patterns in the United States

	Occasional Users	% of Total Consumption	Hardcore Users	% of Tot. Cons.
1989	5,300,000	11.8	3,400,000	88.2
1990	4,600,000	12.6	3,200,000	87.4
1991	4,500,000	15.7	3,000,000	84.3
1992	3,500,000	15.3	3,100,000	84.7
1993	3,300,000	15.9	3,300,000	84.1
1994	2,900,000	14.7	3,200,000	85.3
1995	3,000,000	14.7	3,300,000	85.3

Source: Rhodes (ONDCP), 1997.

Table 6.4 Consumption Patterns of Hardcore Cocaine Users

	Median of SupplyRange	Hardcore Consumption	Cons./ Hardcore User
1989	488.5 MT	430.9 MT	.127 kg
1990	470.5 MT	411.2 MT	.128 kg
1991	472 MT	397.9 MT	.133 kg
1992	496 MT	420.1 MT	.136 kg
1993	413.5 MT	347.8 MT	.105 kg
1994	301 MT	257.2 MT	.08 kg
1995	331.5 MT	282.8 MT	.086 kg

If the number of hardcore users, who account for the vast majority of market demand, has been stable over time, why have estimates of the cocaine supply to the U.S. in Table 6.3 (calculated backward from estimated demand) changed so dramatically over the study period? It is because the operational definition of a hardcore user has changed over the study period. From 1989–1992, each hardcore user was assumed to consume roughly .13 kg of cocaine annually (Table 6.5). From 1993 to 1995, however, the amount consumed by each hardcore user ranged from .08 to .105 kg annually.

Is there reason to expect that the individual consumption patterns of hardcore users would drop significantly after years of relative stability and even small increases? The study authors do not provide an explanation and there is no evidence of this shift elsewhere in the literature. An attempt to reconcile this pattern with price data generates more questions than answers. The underlying rationale for supply side anti-narcotics efforts is that the price of cocaine is an important influence on consumption patterns. If this assumption is indeed true, declines in consumption rates by hardcore users should have been preceded by an increase in cocaine prices for the period 1993–1995. Yet cocaine prices were at an all-time low during this period (see Figure 6.1). Moreover, a noticeable price spike occurred in 1992, when consumption by hardcore users was estimated to be at its highest point! This paradox suggests that there may not be a strong relationship between cocaine price and consumption.

Certainly, there seems little reason to accept the re-definition of hardcore cocaine users from 1993–1995. If we instead assume that annual cocaine consumption by hardcore users remains at the same mean level (.131 kg) as in the 1989–1992 period, the estimated median point of the supply range would be much higher (see Table 6.6). The revised results indicate that

Table 6.5 Revised Cocaine Consumption / Supply Measures

	Hardcore consumption	Total consumption (supply)
1993	432.3 MT	514 MT
1994	419.2 MT	491.4 MT
1995	432.3 MT	506.8 MT

there has been minimal change in the demand for or supply of cocaine to the U.S. from 1989–1995.

The unexplained redefinition of hardcore users creates the misleading impression that the supply-side anti-narcotics measures pursued during this period have successfully reduced the supply of cocaine to the United States. The broader significance of the preceding discussions of cocaine price and consumption data is that such figures are as commonly used to obfuscate than illuminate trends in drug trafficking and use. They provide a valuable demonstration of the point first raised in Chapter One regarding the quality, validity, reliability and comprehensiveness, or lack thereof, of drug-related data.

RETAIL DISTRIBUTION

By the time cocaine reaches the retail market, it will have passed through a number of hands, eventually shifting from control by a multinational DTO to local independent entrepreneurs. For instance, a five hundred kilogram shipment is transported from El Paso, a major distribution hub, to the Chicago area. The shipment is then split into smaller parcels of perhaps fifty kilograms each. These parcels are delivered to major wholesale dealers in the region whom are closely affiliated with the DTO owning the shipment. These major wholesale 'connections' repackage their allotments into 5–10 kilogram lots, which are then distributed to local, independent entrepreneurs (both within Chicago and in nearby cities).

Dealers at this level of the distribution hierarchy are not commonly members of multinational DTOs, but maintain close relationships with their local representatives. These individuals distribute relatively small quantities (kilograms or less) to neighborhood 'connections.' In turn, these high-order retail distributors might supply an affiliated 'crew' of street level dealers directly with small quantities (grams) of cocaine or crack. They might also sell ounce or multi-ounce quantities to freelance retailers (USSC, 1995: 4). In most suburban and rural markets, these freelance dealers are more prominent than ethnic entrepreneurial gangs (NDIC, 2001a: 8). Whatever the case, dealers at this level of the distribution hierarchy are fully separated from the operations of major DTOs.

The distribution hierarchy described here is generic but realistic. It suggests that once cocaine is consolidated near the point of entry, it must pass through four to six levels of the hierarchy until it reaches drug users. It is important to note, however, that the organization and 'length' of distribution channels varies from place to place. The number of transactions between bulk wholesale shipments and retail markets depends on a variety of local factors: the size and order of the market center, its proximity to higher-order centers, and the nature and efficacy of anti-drug police actions.

One certainty is that the closer a transaction is to the retail level, the price per unit rises while the quantities involved decline. Per unit price increases result from the accumulation of transaction costs as well as heightened risks for market participants. At the retail end of the distribution chain, counter-drug efforts are simpler. Exchanges are more open, making tactics like 'buy and bust' more feasible. Moreover, "the absence of third-party control and regulation in these markets makes chicanery, duplicity and violence serious threats to the lead participants (Eck, 1995: 71)." Such occupational hazards mean that street-level distribution appeals to a small segment of the workforce, commonly poor and unskilled minority youth concentrated in urban neighborhoods.

A common perception is that these individuals are high wage earners, but long-term ethnographic studies of street-level distributors suggest otherwise. Venkatesh (2001: 4) concludes that average wages ranged from $6 to $11 an hour. Jacobs (1999: 21) found that the gross monthly income of street distributors of crack cocaine in St. Louis was roughly $2,300, earned from five and a half days of full-time work each week (Jacobs, 1999: 21). This represents *net* earnings of $6–7 an hour, roughly comparable to what street-level dealers could expect to earn in the few licit occupations for which they are qualified. Yet the high risk of death, injury, or incarceration faced by individuals in this line of work diminishes these apparent rewards. Considering that a street seller might conduct hundreds or even thousands of transactions a year, their exposure to risk is enormous (USSC, 1995: 4).

That poor compensation, relative to risk, continues to attract new market entrants reflects the paucity of legal employment options for youth and young adults in at-risk neighborhoods (Dunlap and Johnson, 1997). It is also a reflection of the prevalence and appeal of urban myths associating 'gangsta' drug dealers with expensive cars, clothes, and wads of cash. There are, in fact, few such individuals and they are almost never directly involved with retail drug sales. While most street level dealers are soon disillusioned by their inability to advance into the management of higher-order distribution functions, the myths persist.

The predominant forms of retail cocaine distribution enterprises are freelance operators, small non-gang 'entrepreneurial' groups, and traditional street gangs. Freelancers commonly sell to family, friends, and other 'screened' contacts, and may also sell in open markets. Because they lack the protective advantages of gang-affiliated sellers, they are more subject to intimidation and rip-offs. Small groups of acquaintances often form 'entrepreneurial' gangs that offer a measure of security against competitors, while their small size and often transitory nature make them difficult targets for law enforcement (USSC, 1995: 10). Entrepreneurial gangs are smaller, more cohesive, and less likely to be involved in non-drug related crimes than traditional street gangs. They are not established to promote cultural, social, or neighborhood objectives, but rather to profit from criminal activity. Members are older and have clear, market-defined roles. 'Entrepreneurial' gangs may employ gang-affiliated youth in various capacities, including lookouts, street dealers, or enforcers (Rengert, 1996: 25).

A study sampling over three thousand police departments from across the country reported that perhaps forty percent of drug sales involve traditional youth gang members (Howell and Gleason, 1999: 3). The study concludes that while youth gang involvement is extensive, their intensive involvement is limited to a relatively few jurisdictions. Another study of retail cocaine distribution in two mid-sized suburban cities reached a similar conclusion—that gangs are involved but not dominant (Maxson, 1995: 6). Fragmented, young, and unstable street gangs lack the necessary organization, discipline, and connections to monopolize the distribution of cocaine at any scale beyond their own neighborhoods (Jacobs, 1999: 10).

For successful retail drug transactions to occur, buyers and sellers must meet in a particular location to exchange money and product. To do so, each incurs the risk of apprehension by the police or the theft of goods and money by a criminal third party. In the face of these threats, buyers and sellers can pursue two basic strategies for completing transactions: either sell/buy only to/from 'screened' contacts, or sell/buy to/from anyone. The first option enhances the security of the transaction, but restricts potential opportunities for successful transactions. The second maximizes access and potential transactions but involves greater risk. "How retail sellers and buyers resolve the conflicting demands of access and security has major consequences for the geographical distribution of illicit marketplaces (Eck, 1995: 68)." The prevalence of one form of distribution or another in a particular retail market depends on a variety of factors, including the focus and intensity of local law enforcement efforts, the nature of market demand, settlement density, and even climate.

A 'social network' model of distribution refers to exchanges made between screened buyers and sellers. This model facilitates secure transactions by allowing buyers and sellers to privately signal their accessibility and evaluate exchange partners. These markets have low place attachment because security and accessibility are provided through the network, not through place. They are often widely distributed in space and involve relatively few buyers and sellers (Eck, 1995: 72–74). For cocaine, 'social network' exchanges are commonly managed by 'beepermen' whom buyers contact using phone or pager. 'Runners' are then dispatched to homes, offices, or other designated locations to meet buyers and complete the transaction. Network arrangements of this type maximize privacy and security, and are commonly used to supply relatively upscale clientele located outside inner-city neighborhoods (USSC, 1995: 7).

In the second general model of retail cocaine distribution, exchanges are made in locations used by both buyers and sellers for routine daily activities. Suitable places are those that are familiar to both parties and facilitate communication and exchange. Areas where stranger-to-stranger selling takes place are, therefore, commonly located in and around major thoroughfares and nodes of activity (Eck, 1995: 75). Open-air sales commonly take place in public venues like corners and alleys and serve both walk-up and drive-in buyers. The advantages of such sites include maximum accessibility, minimal overhead, and numerous avenues of escape. Operations often involve security measures like lookouts, decoys, and enforcers to protect the seller from the police, rivals, or theft.

'Routine activity' markets operate most efficiently when sellers can establish a relatively permanent location known to prospective buyers. In this situation, buyers need not waste time and effort searching for a source, and sellers need not increase their risks by actively searching out buyers. To establish a semi-permanent open market, sellers must reach an agreement, either through intimidation or bribery, with place managers (landlords, store owners and employees) at that location. For this reason, open drug markets tend to locate in economically depressed areas, where place managers are often weak or corruptible. Because there are relatively few locations that satisfy needs for both access and security, these markets display high place attachment (Eck, 1995: 75–77).

The threat of law enforcement activities or predatory actions by competitors and consumers can alter traditional location preferences. Rather than choosing places that maximize access to consumers, some dealers may prefer more secure locations where they can monitor and evaluate threats and escape if necessary (Rengert, 1996: 67–9). The use of fixed locations like crack houses can be seen as a choice to maximize security while maintaining a degree of permanence and accessibility. These places are often fortified, have limited access through rear / alley entryways, and seek to limit buyer-seller interaction through slots in bricked or boarded windows (USSC, 1995: 8). While this strategy offers greater security against predatory or opportunistic market participants, it invites scrutiny from law enforcement agencies.

The pattern of cocaine distribution to drug users around a retail marketplace is best modeled using an expansion diffusion process dominated by distance decay effects (Rengert, 1996: 34; Eck, 1996: 20). The concept of distance decay addresses the fact that the total cost of a product to consumers increases with distance from the source. Consumers pay not only the selling price of the good, but also incur costs by moving through additional increments of space. For cocaine consumers, the friction of distance reflects not only tangible expenditures in terms of time or money, but also important intangible costs. These involve the greater uncertainty and risk that result from operating in more distant and less familiar environments. Even in licit retail markets, proximity between sellers and buyers creates a comfortable familiarity that makes accessibility an important location factor, even in those situations where the tangible costs of spatial interaction are negligible (Hanink, 1997: 281–282).

Because consumption declines as costs increase, the effect of distance is to create a spatial demand curve (see Jones and Simmons, 1997: 38–42). The friction of distance gradually increases to the point where costs are prohibitive and spatial interaction ceases. This distance is the range of the good and defines the spatial extent of its market area. Different types of drug markets have different characteristics. Sales locations that cater to drive-in customers will have larger spatial ranges than those serving walk-up neighborhood customers (Rengert, 1996: 72). Retail markets for powder and crack cocaine differ in a number of ways, including the spatial range of sales outlets. Such differences merit further examination.

CRACK COCAINE

Crack is produced by 'cutting' cocaine HCl with baking soda, mixing it with water, and cooking the solution until the water evaporates. This relatively quick and simple process converts the hydrochloride salt into base form, creating a waxy substance that resembles small off-white "rocks." When smoked, these rocks produce a respirable aerosol of cocaine base, delivering within seconds a penetrating and intense euphoria (Jacobs, 1999: 4). These

Table 6.6 Comparison of the Retail Distribution of Powder and Crack Cocaine

Cocaine Powder	Crack Cocaine
Social network market	Routine activity market
Mobile customers (low friction of distance)	Immobile customers (high friction of distance)
Customers not residents of market neighborhood	Customers are residents of market neighborhood
Customer's primary concern is security	Customer's primary concern is price
Higher-order good	Lower-order good
Infrequent purchases	Frequent purchases
Fewer retail sellers	More retail sellers
Typical retail transaction: gram ($50–150) Multiple (5–10) doses	'Rock'–roughly .1 gram ($5–20) Single dose
Larger threshold and range	Smaller threshold and range

very potent individual doses of cocaine can be purchased for as little as $2 to $5, making them popular with heavy users and the poor (Erickson, 1994: 4). Crack was, in fact, developed specifically to expand the cocaine market to include poor customers (Rengert, 1996: 7).

The frictional effect of distance is especially apparent in the organization of retail markets for crack cocaine. Its consumers are generally poorer and less mobile than users of powder cocaine, meaning that they encounter greater friction when moving across space. This sensitivity to distance makes the slope of crack's spatial demand curve much steeper. For this reason, more dealers are needed to satisfy a given spatial demand than would be the case for powder cocaine. Because consumers of cocaine powder have greater mobility, its dealers are less numerous and less likely to be spatially concentrated.

For this reason, the emergence of crack in the mid 1980s dramatically expanded opportunities for street level drug distributors. "Entrepreneurs facilitated access to supplies, offered controlled selling territories, and created entry-level roles in drug selling that required only minimal training and start-up capital (Jacobs, 1999: 4)." Freelance operators, most commonly un- or under-employed inner city youth, account for the majority of retail crack sales. Although groups of these sellers occasionally work together, there is rarely any functional division of labor or a hierarchy of roles. Jacobs (1999: 62) found that "cooperative forms of selling are short-lived, infrequently observed, and generally limited to respecting each other's selling spot." Groups of street level dealers are not sufficiently organized or cohesive to develop more formal or permanent business structures.

Street sellers purchase their inventory from accessible neighborhood 'connections.' These individuals maintain a degree of separation from street retail markets, and are commonly responsible for transforming cocaine powder into crack. This conversion occurs only at downstream distribution stages because of tougher criminal sanctions against the possession of crack cocaine. Risk-averse dealers thus seek to minimize their on-site crack inventories. Customary purchases of crack by street sellers are $50 (1g), $100 (2g), or $250 (quarter-ounce) transactions (Jacobs, 1999: 440). A gram is roughly equivalent to five $20 (at street-level) rocks. Street sellers, therefore, aim to double their initial investment by serving as brokers between drug users and the bottom rung of the wholesale market. In theory, a street dealer could advance his position in the distribution hierarchy by continuously selling inventory and using profits to double the size of wholesale purchases. In practice, this strategy faces significant obstacles, especially in a declining market. As dealers handle larger quantities, the challenge and risk of distributing it escalates. Street sellers often lack sufficient discipline or business acumen to meet these challenges (Jacobs, 1999: 121).

The large margins at this stage of the distribution chain reflect the significant risks faced by market participants. Crack markets are characterized by constant violence and institutionalized duplicity. In contrast to powder users, who commonly rely on a single, secure, primary source, crack users make more frequent purchases from a broader network of potential dealers in relatively visible public spaces (Riley, 1997: 25). Dealers commonly use a variety of 'transactional mediation' schemes in an effort to minimize co-presence with buyers and obfuscate exchanges of money and drugs. These mechanisms include the use of a variety of props, third parties, and cache locations to complete transactions without risking police detection (Jacobs, 1999: 89).

This chapter presents a valuable conceptual framework for describing and evaluating wholesale and retail cocaine distribution in the United States. The marketing of cocaine is a complex process, made comprehensible by the organizing geographic principles adopted in this chapter. The most useful concept for understanding wholesale distribution is central place theory, which offers insight regarding differences in distribution functions, and price and purity characteristics between different markets. Retail distribution is explained using notions of diffusion, spatial interaction, and distance decay. These ideas illuminate the behaviors of different market actors, as well as the organization and orientation of different types of drug markets.

Chapter Seven
Policy Implications

Its analysis presented here of the cocaine trade and the multinational enterprises provides valuable insight for evaluating state policies that influence the industry's business climate. This chapter examines a variety of domestic and international policy concerns related to the drug trade and state responses to it. The geographical perspective applied in this research offers a valuable, yet under-appreciated approach. Because foreign area studies have always been an important component of the discipline, geography is an especially useful means to evaluate the international dimensions of anti-narcotics regimes. The policy discussion presented here is inspired by Peirce Lewis' (1985: 471) presidential address to the Association of American Geographers, in which he argued that the most important task facing geographers is

> to persuade the public about the importance of asking the right geographic questions and getting reliable answers to those questions. If one is to judge from the conduct of American foreign affairs, especially in little-known areas beyond our borders, our success in that enterprise may well have mortal importance. If we persist in sending American armies and American treasures overseas, it is not a bad idea to know where we are sending them—*and why.*

The U.S. is the world's largest cocaine market and consumes tens of billions of dollars of it annually. Federal, state and local authorities have spent hundreds of billions of dollars over the past two decades fighting a 'war' to stem the flow (Economist, 2001d 4; 1997d: 36). Efforts to control the trade rely heavily on supply-side (or source-country) measures emphasizing eradication and interdiction programs. Such efforts involve: minimizing the cultivation of coca; reducing access to precursor chemicals; intercepting shipments of cocaine intermediaries between processing stages; seizing cocaine shipments bound for the U.S.; seizing trafficker's facilities and assets; hindering money laundering operations; and apprehending anyone involved in these activities.

State agencies evaluate the success of such programs using measures like the amount of cocaine seized, the number of traffickers arrested, or the number of processing facilities destroyed. While these figures may reassure the public and provide an illusion of effectiveness, conclusions regarding these efforts are far different when judged on their success in raising the price or reducing the availability of cocaine. Overwhelming evidence suggests that supply-side policies fail to accomplish either goal (Lee, 1999; Drexler, 1997; Holden-Rhodes, 1997; Menzel, 1997; Caulkins, 1994; Filippone, 1994; DiNardo, 1993). It is difficult to find even a trace of optimism for source country control policies outside of official documents. Despite a substantial commitment of resources to increasingly aggressive counter-narcotics operations, the price of cocaine in the U.S. has steadily dropped since the early 1980s while its availability and purity have increased, a sign that supply is more than adequate (USDOJ, 1999, Economist, 1997a: 26). Former ONDCP Director Barry McCaffery commented: "I think we're achieving tactical successes without making an operational difference (see Holden-Rhodes, 1997: 164)."

A 1993 RAND project concluded that even exceptionally successful seizure rates of up to seventy percent have little effect on the cocaine market (Kennedy, 1993: 39). Another study calculated that even if interdiction efforts could intercept half of all cocaine shipments to the U.S., this success would add only about three percent to the final retail price (Painter, 1994: 145). Considering that current interdiction programs intercept perhaps five to ten percent of shipments, they have a minimal impact on cocaine markets at best. Caulkins (1993) argues that interdiction will have a substantial impact on drug consumption "only in the most optimistic of all scenarios." The costs of production for leaf, base, and even refined cocaine HCl represent a small fraction of retail prices. Because massive intervention is required to generate even moderate increases in production costs, such programs have little or no long-term impact on retail prices. Similar findings were reported by DiNardo (1993), who examined the price elasticity of demand for cocaine with respect to the intensification of interdiction efforts

Furthermore, hardcore cocaine users (more than ten times per month) may not respond to price mechanisms aimed at diminishing their use of the drug. These users have a strong preference for the type of high that cocaine delivers and many are addicts. Whether due to preference or dependency, cocaine exhibits very low price elasticity of demand (Riley, 1996: 71). Large price increases cause relatively small declines in demand. Because supply-side interdiction measures produce small, temporary price changes at best, they have been ineffective in reducing cocaine consumption. This fact is reflected by the number of hardcore users in the U.S., which has remained stable at roughly three million for more than a decade according to the Drug Use Forecasting Program (ONDCP, 2000b: 13).

Even if supply side programs could manage to significantly increase retail prices, the changes are bound to be short lived. Higher prices signal traffickers that there are greater potential profits to be gained by *increasing* production and distribution (Friman and Andreas, 1999: 10). Those traffickers able to successfully distribute shipments into the U.S. stand to make even greater profits than before. As traffickers increase production over time, prices decline, eliminating previous gains made by law enforcement efforts. Not only do prices return to the same or lower levels than before, the productive capacity of trafficking organizations is enhanced.

COLLATERAL DAMAGE—FOREIGN AND DOMESTIC

While source country tactics have had little success in restricting the flow of cocaine or reducing its consumption in the U.S., they have turned our national cocaine addiction into a foreign policy headache. Aggressive prohibition efforts and vituperative rhetoric antagonize people and governments of nations throughout Latin America. Regional 'partners' resent regional counter drug efforts, particularly the manner they have been force-fed to date (Holden-Rhodes, 1997: 146). Former Mexican President Ernesto Zedillo spoke for many in the region when he commented:

> The human, social, and institutional costs in meeting [drug] demands are paid for by the producing and transit countries. It is our men and women who die first in combating drug trafficking. It is our communities that are first to suffer from violence, our institutions that are first to be undermined by corruption. It is our governments that are first to have to shift valuable resources needed to fight poverty to serve as the first bulwark in this war (see Smith, 1999: 213).

When the foreign 'war' on cocaine intensified in the mid 1980s, interdiction efforts focused primarily on Caribbean smuggling routes into South Florida. These operations achieved early successes, but were thwarted as traffickers re-routed shipments through 'Pacific' channels. By the end of the decade, a new program concentrating on eradication and interdiction in producer countries was devised. This 'Andean Strategy' was heralded as a major break with past failures, but was really no more than an escalation (and geographical extension) of the same supply-side strategies. The major elements of the strategy were the incorporation of source country militaries Resistance to the militarization of counter-drug operations appeared throughout the region (Holden-Rhodes, 1997: 79–80). Opponents criticized

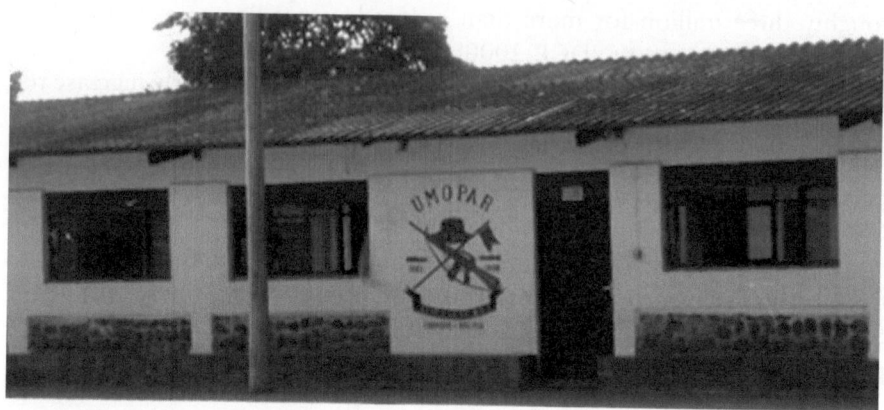

The headquarters of the *Unidad Movil de Partrullaje Rural* in Chimore, Bolivia. This U.S. supported anti-narcotics police unit is responsible for conducting an intensified campaign of forced coca eradication in the Chapare. Tensions between the rural peasantry and UMOPAR units have escalated dramatically in recent years to a series of protests, roadblocks, riots, and fatal conflicts.

the trend for undermining civilian authority and enhancing the position of the military, no minor concern in a historically unstable region with weak democratic traditions. Some saw U.S. drug policy as an infringement on national sovereignty (Laserna, 1995b: 193; Morales, 1992: 169). Others feared that greater military involvement would generate more civil conflict, violence, and human rights violations (Laserna, 1995b: 198; Painter, 1994: 93). The region's governments were unable, however, to resist the combination of U.S. diplomatic pressure and aid incentives. Both U.S. and local military forces have maintained prominent roles in anti-drug enforcement ever since. Currently, the most significant U.S. military role is in Colombia, where the United States is involved in an escalating civil war inextricably tied to drug trafficking (Steinberg, 2000).

An escalation and militarization of counter-drug efforts has also occurred at the U.S.-Mexico border. Here, military personnel are used in a variety of roles to support border law enforcement efforts, including: training, intelligence, operational planning, surveillance, transportation, radar and imaging missions, cargo inspection, and fence maintenance (Andreas, 1998, Harlan, 1997, Kees 1997, Dunn 1996). The adoption of modern war-fighting technologies, (including night-vision equipment, infrared scanning devices, movement sensors, and helicopters) offers further evidence of the militarization of the border–a process that Dunn (1996: 170) argues has "disturbing implications for the human and civil rights of residents and immigrants in the border region."

The militarization of drug prohibition regimes has important but poorly understood implications for the region's long-term peace, security, stability, and prosperity. Nonetheless, it is clear that the cocaine industry cannot be eliminated through aggressive law enforcement in Colombia, Bolivia or Mexico. As a Colombian observer noted, "the struggle against drug trafficking has failed for one simple reason: They are trying to shoot down with bullets the law of supply and demand (Drexler, 1997: 168)." The quote implies an inherent tension between free trade and drug prohibition—a paradox indicating that current policy goals may be incompatible. Policies promoting 'globalization' strengthen DTOs and complicate drug prohibition efforts. Yet both economic liberalization and drug prohibition are actively encouraged by the United States. To continue in pursuit of both is a waste of financial and political capital, and a source of conflict with serious and tangible costs for the Americas.

Treating a domestic social problem as a foreign policy issue has done little to reduce cocaine abuse in the U.S., but has succeeded in transferring some of the political and social costs of the drug 'war' to Latin American and Caribbean nations. This process unfortunately reduces U.S. leverage and international cooperation on a host of important foreign policy matters, including; economic development, democratization and human rights, and the environment. It remains to be seen if the political will exists to address cocaine abuse with domestically oriented demand and harm reduction programs. If not, the U.S. will continue to annoy its neighbors, while millions of cocaine users remain supplied by increasingly sophisticated and resourceful trafficking organizations.

Aggressive and punitive enforcement regimes are also the norm in the U.S. domestic sphere. The focus has typically been on apprehending traffickers and users rather than domestic demand-reduction, education, and rehabilitation programs. For this reason, MacCoun and Caulkins (1996) argue that drug prohibition is itself a major source of drug-related harm. As Ethan Nadelmann, a leading figure in the drug policy reform movement, has observed:

> The failure of most Americans . . . to distinguish between the problems that stem from the misuse of drugs per se and those that stem from drug prohibitionist policies, remains the single greatest obstacle to any significant change in American drug control policies (Nadelmann, 1997: 87).

Drug prohibition, as currently implemented, involves serious social costs that are grossly under-appreciated by policymakers and the public alike. Direct and indirect costs of the domestic 'war' on drugs include: billions of dollars spent annually on drug control; the violence and corruption associated with drug markets; an overburdened criminal justice system, unacceptably high levels of incarceration, the militarization of local police forces, unacceptable infringements on civil liberties, the aggravation of race relations, and *de facto* subsidies of organized crime.

The nature of drug trafficking offenses means that there is no victim to make accusations or provide information. This situation stimulates the development of creative and combative police tactics targeting drug offenders. The procedural rights of Americans have been relaxed in order for such tactics to be implemented, creating the potential for abuse of authority by law enforcement officials. Abuses include illegal searches, harassment of citizens, and the planting of evidence (Rengert, 1996: 88).

> The Fourth Amendment expresses our historical concern regarding state respect for private property. Yet it has been trampled by the demand for greater police authority to rid society of its 'drug menace.' In the wake of this shrinking of Constitutional protection, police agencies have been empowered to make vehicle stops solely on suspicion of illegal activity. Suspicion is all too frequently based on profile characteristics, meaning that the overwhelming number of stops involve minorities and youths. Such an approach helps to explain why minorities constitute more than ninety percent of all prisoners currently incarcerated on drug offenses (Baggins, 1998: 60).

Aggressive retail-level enforcement encourages wholesalers to extend distribution chains in an effort to insulate themselves from these risks. In stimulating a larger, more layered network of dealers, law enforcement activities have unintentionally increased the number of people involved in drug trafficking (Rasmussen and Benson, 1994: 92). Counter-drug efforts targeting domestic distribution are like those in the production and transit zones—dealers engage in effective location (and method) substitution strategies. As enforcement 'barriers' emerge in one place or among a population, traffickers can concentrate sales in other, more hospitable markets. The development of a presence in multiple markets is an important risk-minimization strategy in many businesses.

'OUT-OF THE-BOX' ALTERNATIVES

Andreas (1999b: 94) suggests an explanation for the obstinate determination with which drug prohibition is pursued, despite its obvious limitations:

> It is the very persistence of smuggling that is most critical for sustaining and expanding law enforcement. In other words, even though law enforcement fails to deter the business of smuggling, smuggling also keeps law enforcement in business. This is particularly critical in an era of austerity, shrinking budgets, and antigovernment ideology. In many

countries, the growth of law enforcement is the most striking exception to the general rollback of the state.

A prescient critique was offered in 1972 by the Shafer Commission, an expert panel directed by President Nixon to study the country's drug problem. It concluded that anti-narcotics efforts had (even at that time):

> created ever-larger bureaucracies, ever-increasing expenditures, and an outpouring of publicity so that the public will know that 'something' is being done. Perhaps the major consequence of this . . . has been the creation of a vested interest in the perpetuation of the problem among those dispensing and receiving funds . . . In the course of well-meaning efforts to do something about drug use, this society may have inadvertently institutionalized it as a never-ending project (see Bugliosi, 1996: 263).

The 'never-ending project' matured through the cocaine boom of the 1970s, emerged as a 'war' with international dimensions in the 1980s, and intensified and spread in the1990s. Holden-Rhodes (1997: 174) comments:

> While this approach provides the opportunity for creative rhetoric on the part of politicians so that they can respond to their constituents and argue for large-scale appropriations, it is a 'cop-out,' a failure to respond to the real issues, and a convenient ploy to foist the responsibility and ultimately the blame for their own failure on someone else. The 'war on drugs' is little more than a metaphor crafted primarily for political and propaganda purposes.

Our current national attitude regarding drugs and drug policy is best characterized as a siege mentality. To progress towards a real solution to our drug problem, we must reconsider our single-minded commitment to prohibition. Despite the expenditure of massive effort and resources, policies seeking to stop the flow of cocaine have failed. DTOs are successful business enterprises with considerable resources, and have displayed a great deal of ingenuity and adaptability. It is certain that as long as demand for cocaine exists, DTOs will supply a sufficient quantity to fill the demand. Therefore, drug policies must be developed that minimize the social, political, and economic costs associated with drug trafficking and abuse, in both domestic and international spheres.

The rigorous self-examination and national debate required to elicit this dramatic change of course has not yet begun. As Reuter (1997: 274) notes:

> a society that deliberately averts its eyes from an honest assessment of a massive and frequently cruel intervention that sacrifices so many other

goals for the one desideratum of drug abstinence can scarcely expect to find a well-grounded alternative.

A 'well-grounded alternative' is almost too much to hope for at the present time. What is needed at this time is a comprehensive, open-minded, and public accounting of the costs and benefits of a number of possible alternatives. An incomplete list of alternatives, not mutually exclusive, would include harm-reduction, legalization, decriminalization, de-emphasizing source-country programs, or simply less vigorous enforcement of existing policies. The latter is the least appealing option and not really a policy at all. Rather than finding solutions, it is merely a signal of apathy and defeat.

> The challenge is one of designing and promoting a drug control policy that combines a healthy respect for individual freedom and responsibility with a strong sense of compassion (Nadelmann, 1997: 125).

The favored course among many drug policy reformers is harm reduction—an approach recognizing that some users cannot or will not stop and that drug policies should seek to mitigate the harms these users cause to themselves and others (MacCoun and Caulkins, 1996: 192). Harm reduction does not focus on drug use *per se*, but rather on the harms caused by both drug abuse and prohibition. Proponents argue

> that supply-reduction initiatives are inherently limited, that criminal justice responses can be costly and counterproductive, and that single-minded pursuit of a "drug-free society" is dangerously quixotic (Nadelmann,1998: 113).

A more radical alternative is legalization, which would reduce risks to market participants, causing prices and profits to decline. In doing so, it would reduce opportunities for corruption, violence, and misallocation of resources. For these reasons, Castells (1998: 174) asserts that the legalization of drugs is perhaps the greatest potential threat facing drug trafficking organizations. By diminishing its profitability,

> a legalization strategy would help beleaguered Third-World governments to better cope with assorted threats to national sovereignty and integrity posed by different participants in the drug trade (Lee, 1999: 34).

Opponents of legalization fear that drug abuse will dramatically increase if drugs are not legally sanctioned. This position rests on the assumption that the only obstacle that keeps people from using drugs is fear of apprehension and punishment. Yet other significant obstacles *do* exist: social taboos; religious faith; health concerns; fear of addiction; and simple lack of time or interest. While decreased risk and prices will increase consumption, it is not evident that legalization will result in dramatically higher levels of drug abuse. It is nonetheless a possibility, one that deserves significant research attention–perhaps a trial case. The savings gained from interdiction, apprehension, and incarceration should be applied to education and rehabilitation efforts to minimize the social costs of any increased abuse.

A second general concern regarding legalization is that it sends the message that drug use is acceptable or even encouraged. This need not be the case; it is possible to discourage use while removing legal sanctions at the same time. One need only admit that prohibition has been tried and proven a failure. Legalization is a possible alternative not because the potential abuse of drugs is acceptable, but because the costs of keeping drugs illegal are too great a burden for society to bear any longer.

The cocaine trade and state responses present producer, transit, and user nations with a complex set of economic, political and social problems. The challenges posed by DTOs and drug related harm demand a rational, coherent, and compassionate state reaction. An appropriate response must include both a serious commitment to reducing demand and a comprehensive reconsideration of drug prohibition. This chapter broadens the field of discussion by critically examining current policy regimes influencing the drug trade. The effort to find mutually beneficial solutions to shared problems can only be advanced through such open debate.

Chapter Eight
Conclusions:
Through a Glass, Darkly

The disintegrated functional stages of the cocaine trade, discussed in relative isolation in preceding chapters, are here reassembled. The model of the cocaine industry generated by this research and elucidated in this chapter is schematic and conceptual rather than formulaic. The modeling process applied here is inspired by a catholic view of models that sees them as a structured synthesis of data, rather than as formal laws or equations. This schema is deeply rooted in the economic, social, and political landscapes within which drug trafficking organizations operate. Developing an understanding of this contextual setting is a second important contribution of this research.

This context illuminates the strategic responses of drug trafficking organizations to the opportunities and challenges posed by competitive industrial environments. Models developed by geographers to explain the spatial behavior of multinational firms engaged in licit industries are profitably applied here to the operations of DTOs. By facilitating the development of normative structures to analyze the cocaine industry, they help to bridge the considerable gaps in our understanding DTO behavior. Such gaps result from their illicit and secretive nature and the resulting lack of quality data regarding their operations. The suspect nature of most of the quantitative data currently available justifies the use of the qualitative models presented in this chapter.

Due to the paucity of meaningful quantitative data and the fragmented, context-less character of much of the qualitative information available, the cocaine industry is commonly seen in a 'blur'—poorly understood and poorly addressed by current policies. This project applies corrective 'lenses' to the cocaine trade in an attempt to bring its elements and activities into focus. The 'lenses' used here are a geographical perspective (the variety

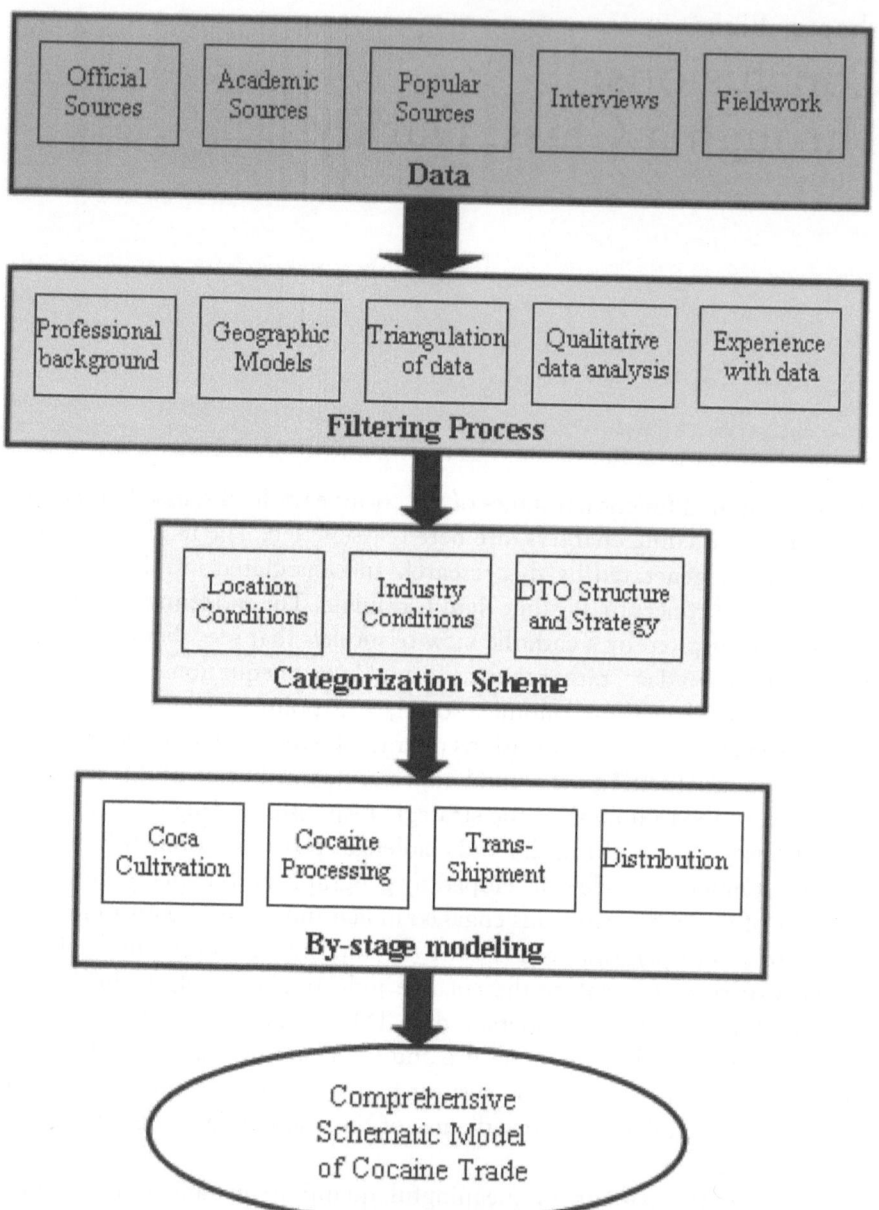

Figure 8.1 Model Development

of geographic models applied in this research) and the process of qualitative data analysis. These 'lenses' must be adjusted to bring pertinent facets of the cocaine industry into focus. Adjustments are made using the author's professional expertise in economic geography and experience with the data. The 'corrective power' of the geographic models applied here varies. They are most effective when applied to specific stages of the production and distribution chain.

For example, a cost-minimization approach to facility location can be usefully employed to analyze coca cultivation and processing of cocaine. The 'optimal' locations for these activities can be determined using traditional variable costs like transportation and wage rates. Cultivation and base processing are heavily oriented toward sources of coca leaf and water. Coca leaves are perishable, bulky, and grown in physically and economically isolated regions. Much of the weight loss in the manufacturing process takes place during the initial conversion. The initial processing stage also use a lot of water and are therefore tied to local water sources. Given the labor-intensity and low value-added in these processes, they are also tied to sources of cheap peasant labor. DTOs involved in the final processing of cocaine HCl prefer locations near sources of both cocaine intermediaries and required precursor chemicals.

Despite a traditional focus on material, labor, and transportation costs, the neoclassical (cost-minimization) approach to location theory is sufficiently flexible to incorporate additional variables and their cost surfaces (Daggett 1968: 58–64). For example, the model developed here could be extended and improved through the development of a 'risk-surface' showing how risk varies from place to place. The minimization of risk is a basic strategy for all drug trafficking organizations at all stages of the value chain. Many expend significant resources collecting and evaluating risk-related intelligence as well as 'purchasing down' risk using bribery. There are, however, difficulties in precisely defining and measuring a concept like risk. It is a function of numerous conditions: the functional orientation of the organization; the degree and nature of market competition; countervailing anti-drug regimes; and the capacity of state actors to enforce them. Moreover, the deficient quality of much drug-related data means that a rigorously quantified risk-surface for the cocaine trade will remain elusive.

Another valuable theoretical 'lens' is enterprise geography, which focuses on the formation of business (especially location) strategy. It emphasizes

> how the geography of corporate strategies is guided by 'internal' long term motivations, accumulated expertise and established corporate structures, and by the 'external' strategies and structures of other

business organizations, especially rivals (but also consumers and suppliers) and by other institutional forms and interest groups (Hayter, 1997: 161).

Dicken (1998) and Glasmeir (2000) are excellent examples in the geographic literature of the use of this approach for understanding firm behavior and organization. Porter (1990) and Dunning (1977) also study firms using similar, explicitly spatial approaches. Enterprise geography contributes to the study of the cocaine trade in a variety of ways, particularly as a tool to evaluate the location substitution strategies successfully employed by DTOs. It is also used to elucidate the industry's transition from a 'Fordist' to a lean production system.

The behavior of firms is a critical element in the development of the theory of competitive advantage, a complex conceptual framework that seeks to explain why certain places succeed in particular industries (Porter, 1990: 29). It is essentially an exploration of how a firm's proximate environment (both geographic and industrial) shapes its competitive success over time. It is a comprehensive approach that tries to integrate many variables, a tactic borrowed and applied in this research.

Central Place Theory and spatial diffusion are valuable conceptual tools for explaining the wholesale distribution of cocaine in the U.S. They are not used in research to develop a rigid, hexagonal system of trade areas (see Dicken and Lloyd, 1990: 25–45). Rather, they are applied as a set of location principles that formalize the complex relationships regarding size, spacing, distribution and service characteristics of cities in an urban hierarchy (Wheeler, et.al., 1998: 153). The wholesale cocaine distribution hierarchy in the U.S. is organized (roughly) according to Christaller's marketing principle. This approach minimizes risk and transaction costs by minimizing the number of transactions required to satisfy a spatially distributed demand. At the retail level, Central Place Theory is no longer relevant. Here, the spatial demand curve and contagious diffusion are more valuable models for explaining the behaviors of suppliers and consumers. Indeed, Eck's (1995a) explicitly geographic typology of retail markets is based in large part on these notions.

The schema used to analyze the cocaine trade is represented graphically in Figure 8.2. The dimensions of the cube represent three intricately inter-woven elements of the industry. The z-axis is the spatial dimension of the model, including all the varied locations where the industry's activities take place. Each place on the z-axis is comprised of sub-regions, each with their own 'local' conditions. Examples include the Yungas and the Chapare in Bolivia and differences between U.S. cities at different levels of the distribution hierarchy. The y-axis represents the functional components of the

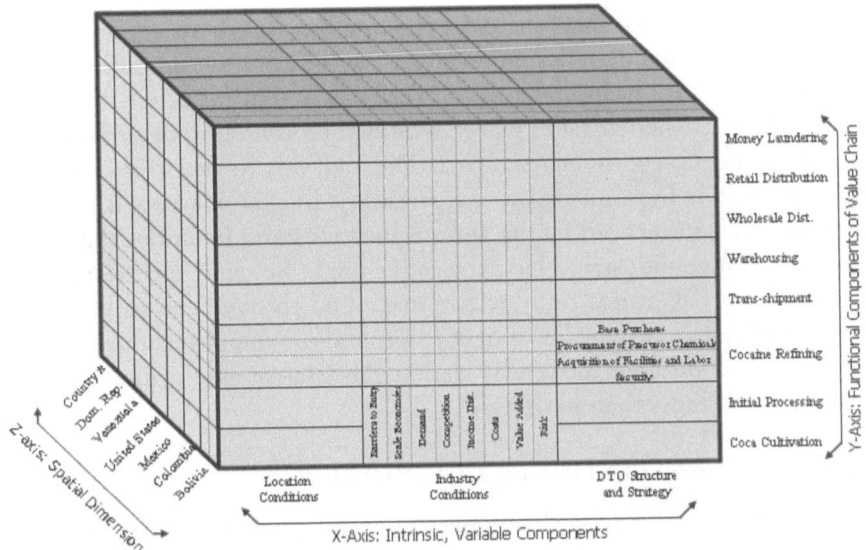

Figure 8.2 A Schematic Representation of the Cocaine Industry

production and distribution chain of cocaine. On the x-axis are the industry's intrinsic, variable elements, organized into three 'master categories.' Due to space constraints, not all sub-categories are included in the graphic, but they are identified in Figure 8.3.

Ideally, a t-axis (time) would be added to figure 8.2. Unfortunately, a feasible technique for graphically representing a fourth dimension has not yet been developed. Regardless, the temporal dimension is critically important to understanding the cocaine trade. Each variable x is dynamic, as is the role and market position of all places z. For example, the industry condition *risk* varies through time in response to changes in the intensity of law enforcement of levels of competition. Similarly, one might contrast the roles played by Peruvian or Dominican DTOs ten years ago relative to today. Peru is much less involved, while the Dominican Republic is much more involved.

The cube can be 'sliced' along any of the three axes, each providing a different perspective for viewing the cocaine industry. The focus can be placed on one location by examining the x and y components corresponding to that place. For example, one might wish to examine how the unique combination of location and industry conditions operating in Bolivia influences the behavior and strategies of Bolivian DTOs. How are these organizations structured? What is the industry's 'footprint' in Bolivia, that is, which functional components are present and/or internationally competitive?

Another way to 'slice' the cube is along the *y*-axis, an approach that emphasizes one functional component of the industry. On might focus on cocaine refining by examining all the variables *x* that influence that stage and all places *z* where it takes place. This method is used to determine how and why a function varies across space. The final way to view this schematic representation is by focusing on one variable *x* to examine how it both influences and is influenced by the various locations and functions that comprise the cocaine industry. This perspective might be used, for example, to evaluate how risk varies both across space and through the value chain. Differences reflect varying levels of capacity and/or commitment to counterdrug efforts in different places, as well as the relative ease of law enforcement in some stages than in others.

LOCATION AND INDUSTRY CONDITIONS

Much of the complexity in the model presented in Figure 8.2 derives from the sixteen intrinsic, variable components of the cocaine industry identified on the *x*-axis. The combined influence of these variables determines the spatial organization of the industry. Their intricate inter-relationships are presented in Fig 8.3. While the network of inter-connections is even denser than portrayed, it should be clear that the strategies and structures of drug

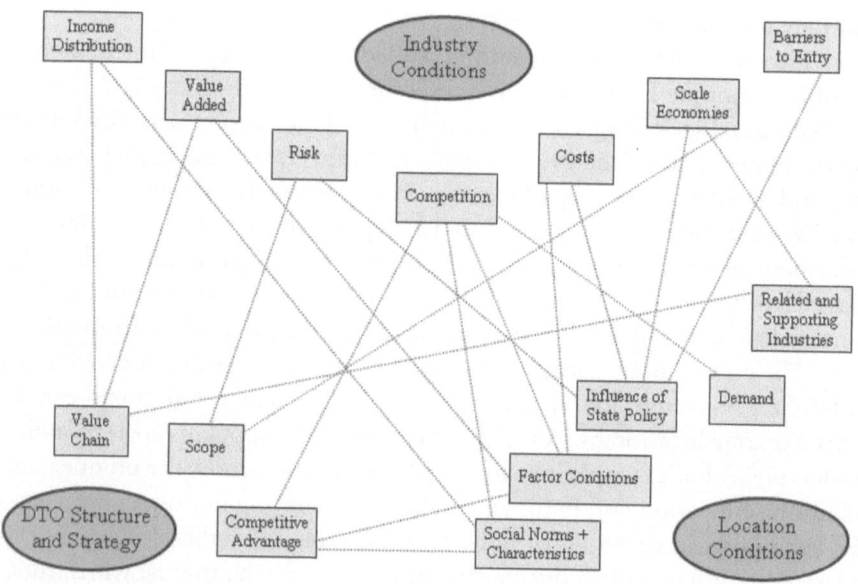

Figure 8.3 Inter-relationships between Master Categories

trafficking organizations are influenced by a variety of industry and location conditions. Significant differences in these variables across space suggest corresponding shifts in the structure and orientation of the industry.

It is tempting to suggest that state counter-drug efforts are the single most important influence the cocaine trade, yet two decades of increasingly aggressive eradication and interdiction programs have had little lasting effect on the availability, purity, price, or consumption of cocaine in the United States. Nonetheless, the degree of enforcement of drug prohibition remains an important variable, differentiated through both space and time, for understanding the industry structure of the cocaine trade. The barriers to spatial interaction presented by various state anti-drug efforts certainly cause risk premiums, transaction costs, and therefore prices to be higher than they would be otherwise. Yet given the price inelasticity of demand for cocaine, it is not clear what effect this has on consumption. There does not seem to be any study that has rigorously investigated the effect of eliminating or relaxing drug prohibition on consumption.

Unfortunately, the model presented here cannot fulfill this worthwhile goal. What it will do is determine what might happen to the industry's price structure, competitive balance, and spatial organization if legal sanctions of cocaine disappeared. Changes in the industry's strikingly unusual price structure would be dramatic. The source of much of the value added to cocaine in the production and (especially) distribution process would disappear immediately. Costs to DTOs for security, bribery, money laundering, and transaction costs would decline precipitously; and firms would therefore command a much smaller risk premium. Prices paid by consumers would reflect these cost savings.

The introduction of legal dispute resolution mechanisms would curtail violence and contribute to dramatically lowered barriers to entry. This would result in greater market competition, further suppressing prices. Cocaine would likely become more pure at the retail level, as firms seek competitive advantage through product differentiation strategies rather than competing on cost. As the product improves and becomes cheaper at the same time, demand for it will likely increase. The exact degree to which demand might rise is currently unknown and worthy of rigorous investigation.

Economies of scale in production would become more important as firms pursue further cost efficiencies. Large, efficient refining facilities would emerge in growing regions, where the entire production process would be concentrated. Refiners would purchase leaves directly from growers who would remain external to an increasingly integrated production system. Coca-cocaine would develop more concrete linkages to the licit economy in source countries, especially the banking, chemical, and transportation sectors. Bolivia and Peru would enjoy some advantages relative to Colombia. Those countries are more stable, produce higher quality leaf, have well organized coca growers, and have plenty of room to expand cultivation. On the other hand, their disadvantages in cocaine refining would remain. Colombian groups enjoy better reputations and downstream connections, superior access to chemical inputs; and higher quality industrial infrastructure, technical expertise, and capital resources. Yet, these advantages would likely diminish over time as Bolivian and Peruvian producers gain experience.

The movement of cocaine to markets would be much simpler and less expensive. Mexican, Dominican, Puerto Rican, Jamaican, Venezuelan groups will likely be cut out of the market, as their expertise in smuggling services would no longer be needed. The distribution chain within the United States would also be organized quite differently, depending on the degree of legalization. To what degree would the distribution of cocaine be decentralized? Would it be available over the counter or restricted to authorized state stores? The latter, more centralized system seems more likely. Either way, many fewer actors would be involved in sales than there are currently.

While state policy is an important influence, the most important variable influencing the cocaine business is demand. The industry has experienced fluctuations in consumer demand, with recent declines in U.S. demand among casual users. Because demand for recreational drugs is more a function of fashion and consumer taste than price, it seems likely that demand will eventually return for cocaine. If demand does increase, it will attract more market entrants, increasing competition and spurring innovation. In the meantime, many cocaine traffickers have diversified in scope by expanding into the production, smuggling, or distribution of methamphetamine, marijuana, and especially heroin, in accordance with their firm-specific competitive advantages. In doing so, they spread risks by gaining exposure to a variety of markets.

Demand must also be evaluated as a location condition. Differences in the nature of demand in each country are reflected in the functional orientation and organization of the cocaine industry there. In Bolivia, for example, there is low domestic demand for cocaine and high demand for coca. The industry is focused on the production of coca and the functionally and geographically linked processing stages of the value chain. On the other hand, the United States has a relatively large domestic demand for cocaine, and very little for coca. Cocaine traffickers here are involved solely in cocaine distribution.

Table 8.1 Location Conditions for Coca Cultivation

- Chronic un- and under-employment in the formal sector, creating excess rural labor
- Soil and climatic conditions favoring coca cultivation
- History of political and social instability
- Large stretches of remote and rugged territory with minimal state presence
- Domestic demand for coca (used in traditional forms)

Table 8.2 Location Conditions for Cocaine HCl production

- History of political and social instability
- Extensive trade and investment linkages with major markets
- Local access to coca inputs and precursor chemicals
- Absence of law enforcement pressure, due either to a lack of capacity or corruption
- Liberalized business environment
- Remote territories characterized by minimal state control
- Large informal economy

Table 8.3 Location Conditions for Cocaine Trans-shipment

- Proximity (in terms of 'economic' distance) to markets
- Liberalized business environment
- A relatively well-developed financial sector for repatriating and laundering profits
- Absence of law enforcement pressure, due either to a lack of capacity or corruption
- Access to natural transportation channels between source countries and markets
- Tradition of commodity smuggling

THE STRUCTURE OF THE COCAINE INDUSTRY AND ITS FIRMS

Like every industry, the cocaine trade is dynamic. Over time, industry conditions, requirements for success, and appropriate business strategies change. One example is the shift from a 'cartel' based structure to one characterized by flexible networks of independent, affiliated firms. Although this trend was

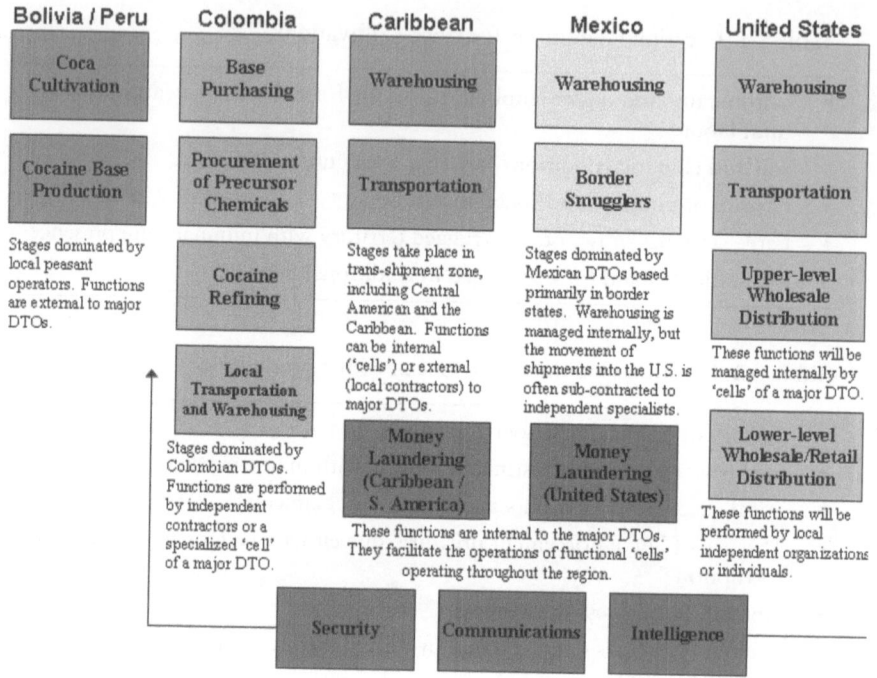

Figure 8.4 An Organizational Structure of the Cocaine Industry and its Firms

already well established, heightened border security since September 2001 has re-emphasized decentralization in the drug trade (Brzezinski, 2002: 26). The use of compartmentalized 'cells' of specialized subcontractors is more important than ever. This sort of flexible network is presented graphically in Fig 8.4. Another worthwhile interpretation of this figure is as a juxtaposition of the y and z axes from the model presented in Figure 8.2.

The production and distribution of cocaine is deeply integrated within the economic and political systems of countries throughout the Americas. The cocaine trade confers unambiguous economic benefits to many parts of Latin America, including foreign exchange, income, and employment. In some countries, the state (or elements within it) has reached a quiet accommodation with DTOs that encourages repatriation of drug wealth (Holden-Rhodes, 1997: 145). Such economic benefits help to explain why authorities are often reluctant to attack the industry at its roots (Lee, 1999: 29).

The specific economic impact of the cocaine trade on any particular place is primarily influenced by the production stage(s) in which it participates. For example, smuggling and marketing of cocaine are more profitable than coca cultivation or cocaine processing. Coca cultivation and initial processing take place in the 'deep' periphery. Even if the physical and economic isolation of these regions could be overcome and suitable alternative sources of income developed, the coca-cocaine industry would persist.

Cocaine traffickers have sufficient resources to match any other economic opportunity that might appear in these regions. By increasing the price they pay for inputs to slightly above what peasants earn from alternative income sources, they raise opportunity costs for farmers, enticing them back into coca cultivation or initial processing. Given the huge revenues gained by DTOs elsewhere in their value chains, they can afford to pay higher input costs without greatly diminishing their profitability.

The failure of state prohibition efforts cannot be explained by a lack of effort, patience, or resources. The explanation lies instead with the nature and organization of the cocaine trade and its component firms, including the mechanisms through which prices at each stage in the chain of production are determined. The industry enjoys many advantages: a product characterized by high value per unit weight, greatly complicating detection and interception of shipments; access to low-cost land, labor, and inputs; an exceptional capacity to make operational adaptations; and strong, sustained consumer demand. This combination of factors provides the cocaine trade with near immunity to supply side control programs of any type or intensity.

Aggressive state responses targeting the drug trade have actually stimulated innovation by criminal organizations by forcing them to be better organized, more efficient, command more sophisticated technology, and also more prone to violence (Friman and Andreas, 1999; Toro, 1995: 1). DTOs have consistently demonstrated exceptional skill at circumventing law enforcement obstacles, developing alternate smuggling routes and innovative smuggling methods, bribing officials, exploiting new sources of precursor chemicals, better concealing processing facilities, or coercing farmers to plant more coca. Successful eradication or interdiction programs only stimulate DTOs to alter either the locations or methods of their operations in order to minimize their impact.

There exist myriad cases where DTOs have shifted operations to areas characterized by relatively minimal law enforcement pressure (the 'balloon effect'). The decline of coca cultivation in Peru and Bolivia in the mid to late 1990s, with a corresponding increase in Colombian cultivation over the same period, provides clear evidence of this phenomenon. Each stage of the production chain can evade law enforcement efforts due to the simplicity and mobility of the processes. Even the least footloose stage, coca cultivation, has many location options. There are vast tracts of suitable and currently unused land in Bolivia, Peru, and Colombia; and Venezuela, Brazil, and Ecuador can serve as alternate suppliers (Riley, 1996: 142). Downstream stages are even more mobile, further hampering anti-drug operations.

The very risk of interdiction losses contributes to cocaine's high price and profitability, because traffickers consider interdiction efforts as merely part of the cost of doing business. They expect losses and maintain sufficient extra capacity in their production systems to make up for moderate levels of interdiction (Riley, 1996: 90). Costs incurred by DTOs from seizure losses are small in relation to potential profits, and market forces entice farmers and refiners to produce more coca and cocaine to make up for seizures. Thus, a kilogram of cocaine HCl seized at a warehouse in Colombia, in a truck along the Mexican border, or on a Bahamian speedboat does not necessarily mean one kilogram less distributed in the U.S.

DTOs produce and distribute cocaine regardless of seizures of shipments, the destruction of processing facilities, or incarceration of traffickers. As long as profits are sufficient to cover costs, business continues. Stable market demand and high profits serve as powerful incentives, stimulating traffickers to pick up where they left off after each successful law enforcement effort. In the short-term, surprise will occasionally allow authorities to catch the industry off guard and inflict significant damage. Yet even in the face of serious short-term pain, traffickers have demonstrated a remarkable ability to make successful long-term adaptations to law enforcement interventions.

INDUSTRY FORECAST

A good test of a model is its ability to develop expectations for the future. The model does so by qualifying the influence of the cocaine industry's important variables and their inter-relationships. Likely changes in these determining variables are identified and evaluated to develop expectations for the industry. Some of the likely scenarios for the cocaine trade are discussed below.

An increased emphasis on border security in the United States since September 2001 presents a familiar challenge to DTOs. In combination with an escalation of international counter-drug operations, increased border security will weed out less capable criminal actors, increase risks for prominent trafficking organizations, and generally accelerate the ongoing process of decentralization and specialization in the industry. Surviving organizations will have to become more sophisticated, focused, and business-like in their approach. The era of flamboyant and excessively violent drug lords and DTOs is over. High-profile organizations like the Arellano Felix brothers,' based in Tijuana, are simply too vulnerable to authorities and competitors alike. The recent elimination of the two most prominent members of that infamous organization, Ramon (killed) and Benjamin (captured), will further encourage the decentralization of Mexican drug trafficking (Economist, 2002b: 43; Sullivan and Jordan, 2002). Indeed, the 'democratization' of drug trafficking can already be seen along the Southwestern border, where many more smaller players are now operating, as evidenced by increasing seizures of very small (1–5 kg) shipments.

The market position of traditionally dominant Colombian DTOs will certainly change as they continue to disengage their cocaine distribution networks in the United States. Not only do they face declining demand for cocaine in the U.S., they also lack competitive advantage at this stage and have steadily lost market share, particularly to Mexican and Dominican distributors. Colombian traffickers will instead supply foreign DTOs that have more capable distribution infrastructure in the United States. Their likely strategic response is to develop markets elsewhere. They have had some success in Europe and will attempt to expand existing markets there. They will also focus on growing markets in countries like Russia, Japan, and China. To do so, they will partner with local criminal groups for distribution. Such partnerships are necessary given the near total absence of Colombian distribution infrastructure in these target countries.

Colombian producers will also focus their resources on the heroin market, which is currently much more lucrative than that for cocaine in the United States (Brzezinski, 2002: 29). Their development of high-purity, smokable heroin has expanded the drug's popularity and market demand. The high purity of Colombian 'white' heroin reflects that country's DTOs' deep historical involvement with the chemical processing of cocaine. The expertise and resources developed over the last few decades from processing cocaine have been successfully transferred to the heroin business. Colombian DTOs will continue their pursuit of process innovations and new products. The introduction of new forms of existing drugs, like smokable cocaine and heroin, has expanded drug markets in the past. Traffickers will again seek to rejuvenate cocaine demand by developing another conveyance, perhaps in pill form. Market diversification, through both geographic and product extension, produces synergies for business organizations. These include both the technology transfers between markets discussed above, as well as the ability to pool risks and stabilize profits (Shepard, 1997: 283–4).

Another likely trend is an increase in coca cultivation and initial processing in Bolivia and Peru, historically the dominant producers at these stages. Uncertainty regarding the direction and implications of Colombia's drug-saturated civil war has already signaled producers in those countries to expand operations. Regardless of the outcome of this conflict, the cocaine trade will adapt operations and carry on business as usual. Even if Colombia ends its civil war, stabilizes economically, re-legitimizes the state, and regains territorial sovereignty (outcomes that seem unlikely at this time), it still would not be able to eliminate drug trafficking. Even if it could, their position would be quickly filled by DTOs from other places. Criminal organizations throughout the region, particularly from Bolivia, Peru, and Venezuela, would be encouraged to enter the market.

Throughout South America, there already exists a popular 'backlash' against both drug prohibition and market-based reforms promoted by the U.S. (Padgett, 2002: 1). Such sentiment is evident in the stunning electoral success of Bolivian coca labor leader and MAS party (Movement Towards Socialism) presidential candidate Evo Morales, who lost a close run-off vote in parliament to former President Gonzalo Sanchez (O'Grady, 2002: A9). Similar attitudes are emerging elsewhere as tough economic conditions again predominate throughout Latin America. Acute fears that Argentina's collapse will spread to other South American countries have already caused capital withdrawal, cutbacks in government spending, bank collapses, jittery financial markets, and recession throughout the region (Economist, 2002d: 34–35). As inflation and unemployment cause living standards to drop, civil and political turmoil ensues (Economist, 2002c: 35). Strikes, road blockades, and violent protests have already been seen Argentina, Peru, and Paraguay (Faiola, 2002; Economist, 2002d: 35).

Severe economic displacement leaves profound impacts on economies and political systems well after the crisis passes. Crises not only elicit new industries, they also can dramatically alter social relations between the state and the public. Latin America's economic ills will certainly encourage drug trafficking, as there are clear historical links between economic crisis and industry growth. These linkages were detailed in the case study chapters, but they are certainly not restricted to those countries. Indeed, the 'Lost Decade' of the 1980s was a region-wide phenomenon which stimulated the growth of cocaine trade. Once established, the industry has been very hard to dismantle. The deepening current crisis bodes ill for future drug control efforts.

In regard to the drug problem in the U.S., former military anti-narcotics intelligence expert J.F. Holden-Rhodes (1997: 175) argues,

> What is needed is detailed, up-to-date information on the structure and performance of drug markets, on the economic, social, and political features of source countries that constrain their responses to the drug problem, and on effects of different policy mixes on the behavior of both markets and countries—in short, the sort of information which is

necessary for a comprehensive and sophisticated analysis which provides policy makers with a better understanding of the complexities they
face and a basis for novel and bold policy making.

This geographical analysis of the cocaine industry will hopefully be
seen as a successful response to that challenge. It demonstrates the discipline's potential to illuminate facts and relationships in a way that forms the
basis of new problem solving paradigms relevant to a variety of vexing social, political, cultural, and economic issues. Geographic tools are applied
not only to countable and measurable physical phenomena, but to an extensive array of human activities and interactions. A geographical perspective
provides the means to organize the disparate sets of facts and relationships
that bear on the cocaine trade, but is equally applicable to other issues.

Bibliography

Acosta, Luis Jaime, 2000. "Colombia Warlord Welcomes U.S. Backed Offensive," *Reuters,* September 28.

Acosta, Luis Jaime, 2000. "Colombia Narco-sub Points to U.S., Russia Drug Tie, *Reuters,* September 13.

Adams, Lisa J. 2000. "Increase in Panama Drug Trafficking," *Associated Press,* April 26.

Allen, Christian M. and Mark deSocio, 2002. "Borderline Nation: Integration and Irredentism in MexAmerica, *Military Review,* October.

Allen, Michael, and Dianne Solis, 1996. "A Mexican Investigator Captures a Druglord," *Wall Street Journal,* April 12: A1.

Anderson, James, 2000. "Caribbean Drug Bust Causes Ripples," *Associated Press,* June 14.

Anderson, John Ward, 2000. "Hard Times Find the Salinas Brothers," *Washington Post Foreign Service,* March 13, 1996: A15.

Andrade, Xavier, 1994. "Drug Trafficking, Drug Consumption, and Violence in Ecuador," in Bagley, Bruce M., and William O. Walker III (eds.) *Drug Trafficking in the Americas,* New Brunswick: Transaction Publishers.

Andreas, Peter, 1998 "The Paradox of Integration: Liberalizing and Criminalizing Flows across the U.S.-Mexican Border," in Wise, Carol (ed.) *The Post-NAFTA Political Economy: Mexico and the Western Hemisphere,* University Park: The Pennsylvania State University Press.

Andreas, Peter, 1999. "When Policies Collide: Market Reform, Market Prohibition, and the Narcotization of the Mexican Economy," in Friman, Richard H. and P. Andreas (eds.), *The Illicit Global Economy and State Power,* Boulder: Rowman &Littlefield Publishers, Inc., pp. 125–141.

Andreas, Peter, 1999. "Smuggling Wars: Law Enforcement and Law Evasion in a Changing World," in *Transnational Crime in the Americas,* Farer, Tom (ed.), New York: Routledge. pp. 85–98.

Andreas, Peter, 2000. *Border Games: Policing the U.S. Mexico Divide,* Ithaca: Cornell University Press.

Antezana, Oscar, 1997. *Bolivia's Coca-Cocaine Sub-Economy in 1996: A Computer Model,* USAID, Bolivia.

Associated Press, 2000. "Cocaine, Heroin Widely Available," March 22.

Associated Press, 2000. "DEA: Cocaine Production Grows," January 18.

Associated Press, 2000. "Study Finds Drug War Targets Blacks," June 8.

Axelsson, Bjorn, and Geoffrey Easton, 1992. Industrial Networks: a New View of Reality, London: Routledge.

Baggins, David Sadofsky, 1998. *Drug Hate and the Corruption of American Justice,* Westport, CT: Praeger.

Bagley, Bruce M., 1997. *Drug Trafficking Research in the Americas: An Annotated Bibliography,* Miami: North-South Center.

Bajak, Frank, 1999. "U.S. Help May Hurt Colombia," *Associated Press,* September 14.

Bajak, Frank, 2000. "Colombia Coca Crops Still Thriving," *Associated Press,* February 21.

Barnes, T., 1988. a reply to "Lets Keep Economics and Geography in Economic Geography," *The Canadian Geographer,* Vol. 32: 347–350.

Barnes, Trevor J., 2001 "Retheorizing Economic Geography: From the Quantitative Revolution to the Cultural Turn," *Annals of the Association of American Geographers,* Vol. 91(3): 546–565.

Beers, Rand, 2000. "Remarks before Senate Foreign Relations Committee," Feb. 25, www.state.gov>.

Berg, Lawrence and Juliana Mansvelt, 2000. "Writing In, Speaking Out: Communicating Qualitative Research Findings," in Hay, Iain (ed.) *Qualitative Research Methods in Human Geography,* Oxford University Press.

Blouet, Brian W. and Olwyn M. Blouet, 1993. *Latin America and the Caribbean: A Systemic and Regional Survey,* New York: John Wiley & Sons, Inc.

Bowden, Mark, 2001. *Killing Pablo,* New York: Atlantic Monthly Press.

Bradshaw, Matt and Elaine Stratford, 2000. "Qualitative Research Design and Rigor," in Hay, Iain (ed.) *Qualitative Research Methods in Human Geography,* Oxford University Press.

Brzezinski, Matthew, 2002. "Re-engineering the Drug Business," The New York Times Magazine, June 23: 24–55.

British Broadcasting Corporation, 2002. "FARC Demands Bilateral Truce," January 24.

Brohman, John, 1996. "Postwar Development in the Asian NICs: Does the Neoliberal Model Fit Reality?" *Economic Geography,* Vol. 72, pp. 107–130.

Bugliosi, Vincent T., 1996. *The Phoenix Solution,* Beverly Hills: Dove Books.

Cabrera Lemuz, Adalid, 2000. "Bolivia Pledges Coca Destruction," *Associated Press,* May 22.

Castells, Manuel, 1998. "The Perverse Connection: The Global Criminal Economy," in *End of Millennium.*

Castells, Manuel, 2000. The Rise of Network Society, Oxford: Blackwell Publishers.

Caulkins, Jonathan P., Gordon Crawford, and Peter Reuter, 1993. "Simulation of Adaptive Response: A Model of Drug Interdiction," *Mathematical and Computer Modeling,* Vol. 17, No. 2, pp. 37–52.

Caulkins, Jonathan P., 1994. "What is the Average Price of an Illicit Drug?" *Addiction,* Vol. 89, No. 7, pp. 815–819.

Caulkins, Jonathan P. 1994. "Evaluating the Effectiveness of Interdiction and Source Country Control Policies," *Economics of the Narcotics Industry,* Conference Proceedings, Dept. of State and the Central Intelligence Agency.

Caulkins, Jonathan P., 1995. "Domestic Geographic Variation in Illicit Drug Prices," *Journal of Urban Economics*, Vol. 37, pp. 38–56.

Caulkins, Jonathan, and Peter Reuter, 1996. "The Meaning and Utility of Drug Prices," *Addiction*, Vol. 91, No. 9, pp 1261–1264.

Caulkins, Jonathan P., 1997. "Modeling the Domestic Distribution Network for Illicit Drugs," *Management Science*, Vol. 43, No. 10, pp. 1364–1371.

Caulkins, Jonathan P., 1997. "Is Crack Cheaper than (Powder) Cocaine?" *Addiction*, Vol. 92, No. 11, pp. 1437–1443.

Castaneda, Jorge G., 1995. *The Mexican Shock*, New York: The New Press.

Caves, R.E., 1971. "International Corporations: the Industrial Economics of Foreign Investment," *Economica*, Vol. 38, pp. 1–27.

Charmaz, Kathy, 2000. "Grounded Theory: Objectivist and Constructivist Methods," in Denzin and Lincoln, eds. *Handbook of Qualitative Research*. Thousand Oaks: Sage Publications.

Chorley, Richard J. and Peter Haggett, 1967. *Models in Geography*. Methuen & Co. Ltd.

Clark, Gordon, 1998. "Stylized Facts and Close Dialogue: Methodology in Economic Geography, "Annals *of the Association of American Geographers*. 88(1), pp. 73–87.

Clawson, David L., 2000. *Latin America and the Caribbean: Lands and People*, Boston: McGraw Hill.

Clawson, Patrick L. and Rensselaer W. Lee III, 1996. *The Andean Cocaine Industry*, New York: St. Martin's Press.

Conkling, Edgar C., and James E. McConnell, 1981. "Toward an Integrated Approach to the Geography of International Trade," in *The Professional Geographer*, Vol. 33, No. 1, pp. 16–25.

Daggett, Stuart, 1968. "The System of Alfred Weber," in R.H.T. Smith, E.J. Taaffe, and L.J. King (eds.), *Readings in Economic Geography: The Location of Economic Activity*, Chicago: Rand McNally, pp. 58–64.

Dear, Michael, 1988. "The Postmodern Challenge: Reconstructing Human Geography," *Transactions of the Institute of British Geographers*, No. 13, pp 262–274.

Del Casino, Vincent J., Andrew J. Grimes, Stephen P. Hanna, and John Paul Jones III, 2000. "Methodological Frameworks for the Geography of Organizations," *Geoforum*, Vol. 31, No. 4, pp. 523–538.

Dewey, John, 1927. "Imperialism is Easy," *The New Republic*, March 23.

Dicken, Peter, 1992. "International Production in a Volatile Regulatory Environment: The Influence of National Regulatory Policies on the Spatial Strategies of Transnational Corporations," in Bryson, John, Nick Henry, David Keeble, and Ron Martin (eds.), *The Economic Geography Reader*, Chichester, John Wiley & Sons, pp. 115–120.

Dicken, Peter, 1994. "Global-Local Tensions: Firms and States in the Global Space-Economy," *Economic Geography*, Vol. 70, pp. 101–128.

Dicken, Peter, 1998. *Global Shift: Transforming the World Economy*, New York: The Guilford Press.

Dicken, Peter and Lloyd, Peter E., 1990, *Location in Space: Theoretical Perspectives in Economic Geography*, New York: Harper Collins.

DiNardo, John, 1993. "Law Enforcement, The Price of Cocaine, and Cocaine Use," *Mathematical and Computer Modeling,* Vol. 17, No. 2, pp. 53–64.

Dombrey-Moore, Bonnie, Susan Resetar, and Michael Childress, 1994. *A System Description of the Cocaine Trade,* Santa Monica: RAND.

Drexler, Robert W., 1997. *Colombia and the United States: Narcotics Traffic and a Failed Foreign Policy,* London: MacFarland & Company, Inc.

Dunlap, Eloise and Bruce D. Johnson, 1992. "The Setting for the Crack Era: Macro Forces, Micro Consequences," *Journal of Psychoactive Drugs,* Vol. 24, No. 4, pp. 307–321.

Dunn, Timothy J., 1996. *The Militarization of the U.S.-Mexico Border, 1978–1992,* Austin: Center for Mexican American Studies.

Dunning, John H., 1977. "Trade, Location of Economic Activity and the MNE: A Search for an Eclectic Approach," in B. Ohlin, P.O. Hesselborn and P.M. Wijkman (eds) *The International Allocation of Economic Activity,* MacMillan, London, pp. 395–418.

Eck, John E., 1995. "A General Model of the Geography of Illicit Retail Marketplaces," in Eck, John E. and David Weisburd (eds.) *Crime and Place,* Monsey, NY: Criminal Justice Press.

Eck, John E., 1995. "What Do Those Dots Mean? Mapping Theories with Data," in Eck, John E. and David Weisburd (eds.) *Crime and Place,* Monsey, NY: Criminal Justice Press.

The Economist, 1993. "Mexico: Fighting Drugs," Aug. 7: 39–40.

The Economist, 1995. "The Mexican Connection," Dec. 16: 39–40.

The Economist, 1997. "Mexico, America, and Drugs," Mar. 29: 25–26.

The Economist, 1997. "Honduras: A Space for Drugs," Mar. 29: 50.

The Economist, 1997. "Neighbours," Mar. 29: 25–26.

The Economist, 1997 "Mexico's Drug Menace: Poison across the Rio Grande," Nov. 15: 36–38.

The Economist, 1997. "The Drug Mob Fights Back," Dec. 13: 29.

The Economist, 1998. "Drugs, Latin America, and the United States," Feb. 7: 35–36.

The Economist, 1998. "Coca, a Bolivian Crop," Mar. 7: 33.

The Economist, 1999. "Colombia in the Long Shadow of War," July 17: 31–32.

The Economist, 2000. "Colombia: A New War," Jan. 15: 34.

The Economist, 2000. "Colombia: War and Peace," Feb. 26: 46.

The Economist, 2000. "A Muddle in the Jungle," Mar. 4: 17–18.

The Economist, 2000. "The Andean Coca Wars," Mar. 4: 23–25.

The Economist, 2000. "Dealing with Colombia's Death Squads," April 8: 35–36.

The Economist, 2000. "A Tidal Wave of Drugs," June 24: 42.

The Economist, 2000. "Few Friends Left for Colombia's Peace Talks," December 16: 39–40.

The Economist, 2001. "Coca's Second Front," January 6: 30–31.

The Economist, 2001. "Drugs, War and Democracy: A Survey of Colombia," April 21: 1–16.

The Economist, 2001. "The Struggle to Eliminate a Much-Loved Andean Shrub," May 26: 35–6.

The Economist, 2001. "A Survey of Illegal Drugs," July 28: 1–16.

The Economist, 2001. "Drowning in Cheap Coffee," September 29: 43–44.

The Economist, 2002. "Haiti–Where Racketeers Rule," February 2: 34.

The Economist, 2002. "The End of the Arellanos," March 16: 43.

The Economist, 2002. "Argentina's Collapse: Return to the Dark Ages," March 16: 35–6.

The Economist, 2002. "South America's Financial Crisis," June 29: 34–5.

Ehlers, Scott, 1999. *Policy Briefing: Asset Forfeiture,* Washington DC: The Drug Policy Foundation.

Erfani, Julie A., 1995. *The Paradox of the Mexican State: Rereading Sovereignty from Independence to NAFTA,* Boulder: Lynne Rienner Publishers.

Erickson, Patricia G., Edward M. Adlaf, Reginald G. Smart, and Glenn F. Murray, 1994. *The Steel Drug: Cocaine and Crack in Perspective,* New York: Lexington Books.

Esparza, Adrian X., and Andrew J. Krmenec, 1996. "The Spatial Markets of Cities Organized in a Hierarchical System," *Professional Geographer,* Vol. 48, No. 4, pp. 367–378.

Faiola, Anthony, 2002. "Economic Crisis Swells in South America," *Washington Post,* Aug 1.

Farer, Tom, 1999. "Fighting Transnational Organized Crime: Measures Short of War," in Farer (ed.) Transnational Crime in the Americas, New York: Routledge. Pp. 245-296.

Faul, Michelle, 2000. "Haiti Labeled as Drug State," *Associated Press,* May 22.

Ferrerya, Aleida and Renata Segura, 2000. "Examining the Military in the Local Sphere Colombia and Mexico, *Latin American Perspectives,* Vol. 27, No. 2, pp. 18–35.

Filippone, Robert, 1994. "The Medellin Cartel: Why We Can't Win the Drug War," *Studies in Conflict and Terrorism,* Vol. 17, pp. 323–344.

Flaherty, Susan, 2001. "The Bolivian Reality," *Towson,* Vol. 5, No. 2, pp. 22–25.

Forbes, Dean, 2000. "Reading Texts and Writing Geography," in Hay, Iain (ed.) *Qualitative Research Methods in Human Geography,* Oxford University Press.

Forero, Juan, 2001. "Judge in Colombia Halts Spraying of Crops," *New York Times,* July 30.

Friman, H. Richard, 1996. *NarcoDiplomacy: Exporting the U.S. War on Drugs,* Ithaca: Cornell University Press.

Friman, H. Richard and Peter Andreas, 1999. "International Relations and the Illicit Global Economy," in *The Illicit Global Economy and State Power,* Lanham, MD: Rowman & Littlefield Publishers.

Gamarra, Eduardo A., 1999. "Transnational Criminal Organizations in Bolivia," in *Transnational Crime in the Americas,* Farer, Tom (ed.), New York: Routledge. pp. 171–191.

Gedda, George, 1998. "Corruption Clouds Anti-Drug Efforts," *Associated Press,* July 18.

Gedda, George, 1999. "Colombia Coca Output Seen Rising," *Associated Press,* October 6.

Gedda, George, 2000. "CIA: Colombia Cocaine Production Up," *Associated Press,* February 15.

Glasmeier, Amy K., 2000. *Manufacturing Time: Global Competition in the Watch Industry, 1795–2000,* New York: The Guilford Press.

Goodchild, Michael F., 1992. "Analysis," in Abler, R., Marcus, M., and J. Olson (eds.), *Geography's Inner Worlds,* New Brunswick: Rutgers University Press, pp. 138–162.

Gray, Mike, 1998. *Drug Crazy,* New York: Random House.

Griffith, Ivelaw Lloyd, 1997. *Drugs and Security in the Caribbean,* University Park, Pennsylvania: Penn State University Press.

Guggenheim, Ken, 2000. "U.S. Braces for Rise in Peru Coca," *Associated Press,* December 23.

Haig, R.M., 1926. Toward an Understanding of the Metropolis, *Quarterly Journal of Economics,* Vol. 40, pp. 421–33.

Hagstrom, Peter, 2000. "Relaxing the Boundaries of the Firm," in Birkinshaw and Peter Hagstrom (eds.) The Flexible Firm: Capability Management in Network Organizations, Oxford University Press. Pp. 201–212.

Hakansson, Hakan and Jan Johansen, 1993. "The Network as a Governance Structure," in Grabher, Gernot (ed.) The Embedded Firm: On the Socioeconomics of Industrial Networks, London: Routledge. Pp. 35–51.

Hall, Kevin G., 2000. "Drug War Sending Coca Leaf Prices Upward in the Andes," *Miami Herald,* October 5.

Hanink, Dean M., 1994. *The International Economy: A Geographic Perspective,* New York: John Wiley & Sons, Inc.

Hanink, Dean M., 1997. *Principles and Applications of Economic Geography,* New York: John Wiley & Sons.

Harvey, David, 1969. *Explanation in Geography,* London: Edward Arnold.

Harvey, David, 1984. "On the Present Condition of Geography: An Historical Materialist Manifesto," *The Professional Geographer,* Vol. 36(1), pp. 1–11.

Hay, Colin and David Marsh, 2000. Demystifying Globalization, New York: St. Martin's Press.

Hays, Tom, 2000. "Army Colonel to Plead Guilty," *Associated Press,* April 4.

Hayter, Roger, 1997. *The Dynamics of Industrial Location,* New York: John Wiley & Sons.

Healy, Kevin, 1994. "Recent Literature on Drugs in Bolivia," in Bagley, Bruce M., and William O. Walker III (eds.) *Drug Trafficking in the Americas,* New Brunswick: Transaction Publishers.

Herod, Andrew, Susan M. Roberts, and Gearoid O Tuathail, 1998. An Unruly World?: Globalization, Governance, and Geography, London: Routledge.

Holden-Rhodes, J.F., 1997. *"Sharing the Secrets: Open Source Intelligence and the War on Drugs,* Westport, CT: Praeger.

Holland, Jesse J., 2000. "Puerto Rico Called Drug Pipeline," *Associated Press,* May 9.

Howell, James C. and Debra K. Gleason, 1999. "Youth Gang Drug Trafficking," Juvenile Justice Bulletin, U.S. Dept. of Justice.

International Crime Threat Assessment, 2000. *President's International Crime Control Strategy,* Interagency Working Group.

Jacobs, Bruce A., 1999. *Dealing Crack: The Social World of Streetcorner Selling,* Boston: Northeastern University Press.

Jones, Ken and Jim Simmons, 1990. *The Retail Environment,* London: Routledge.

Kay, Cristobal, 1993. "For a Renewal of Development Studies: Latin American Theories and Neoliberalism in the Era of Structural Adjustment," *Third World Quarterly,* Vol. 14, No. 4, pp. 691–702.

Kennedy, Michael, Peter Reuter, and Kevin Jack Riley, 1993. *A Simple Economic Model of Cocaine Production,* Santa Monica: RAND.

Kitchin, Rob and Nicholas J. Tate, 2000. *Conducting Research into Human Geography: Theory, Methodology and Practice,* London: Prentice Hall.

Klein, Herbert S., 1986. "Coca Production in the Bolivian Yungas," in *Drugs in the Western Hemisphere: An Odyssey of Cultures in Conflict,* 1996. Wilmington: SR Books. pp. 22–34.

Klein, Herbert S., 1992. *Bolivia: The Evolution of a Multi-Ethnic Society,* Oxford: Oxford University Press.

Kolars, John and John Nystuen, 1974. *Human Geography: Spatial Design in World Society,*

Kotler, Jared, 2000. "Colombia Rebels Fight Drug Effort," *Associated Press,* June 29.

Krauss, Clifford, 2000. "Bolivia Wiping Out Coca, at a Price," *New York Times,* October 23.

Krmenec, Andrew J. and Adrian X. Esparza, 1999. "City Systems and Industrial Market Structure," *Annals of the Association of American Geographers,* Vol. 89(2), pp. 267–289.

Krooth, Richard, 1995. *Mexico, NAFTA and the Hardships of Progress,* London: McFarland & Company, Inc.

La Botz, Dan, 1995. *Democracy in Mexico: Peasant Rebellion and Political Reform,* Boston: South End Press.

Laserna, Roberto, Vargas, Gonzalo V., and Juan A. Torrico, 1995. *La Estructura Industrial del Nacrotrafico en Cochabamba,* Cochabamba: UNDCP-PNUD.

Laserna, Roberto, 1995. *Coca Cultivation, Drug Traffic and Regional Development in Cochabamba, Bolivia,* Unpublished Dissertation.

Laserna, Roberto, 1997. *20 (Mis)Conceptions on Coca and Cocaine,* La Paz: Clave.

Laulajainen, Risto, 1995. "Corporate Geography Relaunched," *Geographical Review of Japan,* Vol. 68, No. 2, pp. 185–197.

Lee, Rensselaer W. III, 1999. "Transnational Organized Crime: An Overview" in *Transnational Crime in the Americas,* Farer, Tom (ed.), New York: Routledge. pp. 1–38.

Lemuz, Adalid Cabrera, 2000. "Bolivia Pledges Coca Destruction," *Associated Press,* May 22.

Lewis, Peirce, 1985. "Beyond Description," *Annals of the Association of American Geographers,* Vol. 75(4), pp. 465–477.

MacCoun, Robert and Jonathan Caulkins, 1996. "Examining the Behavioral Assumptions of the National Drug Control Strategy," in Bickel, Warren K. and Richard J. DeGrandpre (eds.) *Drug Policy and Human Nature,* New York: Plenum Press, pp. 177–197.

MacCoun, Robert and Peter Reuter, 1998. "Drug Control," in Tonry, Michael (ed.) *The Handbook of Crime and Punishment,* New York: Oxford University Press.

MacGregor, Felipe E. (ed.), 1993. *Coca and Cocaine: An Andean Perspective,* London: Greenwood Press.

Maingot, Anthony P., 1994. "The Drug Trade in the Caribbean: Policy Options," in Bagley, Bruce M., and William O. Walker III (eds.) *Drug Trafficking in the Americas,* New Brunswick: Transaction Publishers.

Maingot, Anthony P., 1999. "The Decentralization Imperative and Caribbean Criminal Enterprises," in *Transnational Crime in the Americas,* Farer, Tom (ed.), New York: Routledge. pp. 143–170.

Malamud-Goti, Jaime, 1992. "Reinforcing Poverty: The Bolivian War on Cocaine," in McCoy, Alfred W. and Alan A. Block (eds.) *War on Drugs: Studies in the Failure of U.S. Narcotics Policy,* Boulder: Westview Press.

Maxson, Cheryl L., 1995. "Street Gangs and Drug Sales in Two Suburban Cities," *National Institute of Justice Research in Brief,* U.S. Dept. of Justice.

McCaffery, Barry R., 1998. "Organizing Drug Control Efforts along the Southwest Border," *Office of National Drug Control Policy,* www.whitehousedrug>policy.gov.

McCaffery, Barry R., 1998. "Illegal Drugs: A Common Threat to the Global Community," *United Nations Chronicle,* www.whitehousedrugpolicy.gov.

McCaffery, Barry R., 1999. "Congressional Testimony." www.usinfo.state.gov/topical/global/drugs/ondcp

McFarren, Peter, 2000. "Farmers Block Key Bolivian Road," *Associated Press,* April 17.

McGirk, Tim, 1999. "A Carpet of Cocaine," *Time,* August 9: 51.

Menzel, Sewall H., 1996. *Fire in the Andes: U.S. Foreign Policy and Cocaine Politics in Bolivia and Peru,* New York: University Press of America, Inc.

Menzel, Sewall H., 1997. *Cocaine Quagmire: Implementing the U.S. Anti-Drug Policy in the North Andes-Colombia,* New York: University Press of America, Inc.

Miller, J Mitchell and Lance H. Selva, 1994. "Drug Enforcement's Double-Edged Sword: An Assessment of Asset Forfeiture Programs," *Justice Quarterly,* Vol. 11, No. 2, pp. 313–335.

Mora, Frank O., 1994. "Paraguay and International Drug Trafficking," in Bagley, Bruce M., and William O. Walker III (eds.) *Drug Trafficking in the Americas,* New Brunswick: Transaction Publishers.

Morales, Waltraud Queiser, 1992. *Bolivia: Land of Struggle,* Boulder: Westview Press.

Mortimer, Golden W, 1901. "The History of Coca: The Divine Plant of the Incas," *Drugs in the Western Hemisphere: An Odyssey of Cultures in Conflict,* 1996. Wilmington: SR Books. pp. 2–8.

Müller, German Costas, 1997. *Coca-Cocaina: ¿Conflicto Sin Solucion?,* La Paz: Soi Pa Ltda.

Mulligan, Gordon F., 1984. "Agglomeration and Central Place Theory: A Review of the Literature," *International Regional Science Review,* Vol. 9, No. 1, pp, 1–42.

Nadelmann, Ethan A., 1997. "Thinking Seriously About Alternatives to Drug Prohibition," in McShane, Marilyn and Frank P. Williams III (eds.) *Drug Use and Drug Policy,* New York: Garland, pp. 269–316.

Nadelmann, Ethan A., 1998. "Commonsense Drug Policy," *Foreign Affairs,* Vol. 77, No. 1, pp.111–126.

National Drug Intelligence Center, 2001. *National Drug Threat Assessment,* at www.usdoj.gov/ndic/pubs/647/cocaine.

National Drug Intelligence Center, 2001. *Illinois Drug Threat Assessment,* at
www.usdoj.gov/ndic/pubs/652/cocaine.

National Drug Intelligence Center, 2001. *Indiana Drug Threat Assessment,* at
www.usdoj.gov/ndic/pubs/660/cocaine.

National Drug Intelligence Center, 2001. *Ohio Drug Threat Assessment,* at
www.usdoj.gov/ndic/pubs/658/cocaine.

National Institute on Drug Abuse, 2000. *Epidemiological Trends in Drug Abuse,* at
www.nida.nih.gov

Observatoire Geopolitique des Drogues, 1996. *The Geopolitics of Drugs,* 1996
Edition, Boston: Northeast University Press.

Office of the President of the Republic, 1989. *The Fight Against the Drug Traffic in
Colombia,* Colombia.

Office of National Drug Control Policy, 2000. *Estimation of Cocaine Availability,
1996–1999.* Washington D.C.: Office of Programs, Budget, Research, and
Evaluations.

Office of National Drug Control Policy, 2000. *What America's Users Spend on
Illegal Drugs 1988–1998.* at whitehousedrugpolicy.com

Office of National Drug Control Policy, 2001. *Pulse Check: Trends in Drug Abuse.*
at www.ondcp.gov.

O'Connor, K., 1987. "The Location of Services Involved with International Trade,"
Environment and Planning A, Vol. 19, pp. 687–700.

O'Grady, Mary Anastasia, 2002. "U.S. Policy Fuels Populism in South America,"
The Wall Street Journal, July 12: A9.

Ó hUallacháin, Breandán, 1993. "Industrial Geography," *Progress in Human
Geography,* Vol. 17, No. 4, pp. 548–555.

Oppenheimer, Andres, 1996. *Bordering on Chaos,* Boston: Little, Brown and
Company.

Otero, Gerardo, 1996. "Neoliberal Reform and Politics in Mexico: An Overview,"
in Gerardo Otero (ed), *Neoliberalism Revisited: Economic Restructuring and
Mexico's Political Future,* Boulder: Westview Press.

Padgett, Tim and Elaine Shannon, 2001. "The Border Monsters," *Time,* June 11.

Padgett, Tim, 2002. "Taking the Side of the Coca Farmer," *Time,* August 1.

Painter, James,1994. *Bolivia & Coca: A Study in Dependency,* Boulder: Lynne
Rienner Publishers.

Passas, Nikos, 2001. "Globalization and Transnational Crime: Effects of
Criminogenic Asymmetries, in Williams, Phil and Dimitri Vlassis (eds).
Combating Transnational Crime: Concepts, Activities and Responses.
London: Frank Cass. Pp. 22–56.

Porter, Michael, 1985. *Competitive Advantage: Creating and Sustaining Superior
Performance,* New York: The Free Press.

Porter, Michael, 1990. *The Competitive Advantage of Nations,* New York: The Free
Press.

Ramos, Reyes, 1995. *An Ethnographic Study of Heroin Abuse by Mexican
Americans in San Antonio, TX,* Austin: Texas Commission on Alcohol and
Drug Abuse.

Rasmussen, David W. and Bruce L. Benson, 1994. *The Economic Anatomy of a
Drug War,* Lanham, MD: Rowman & Littlefield.

Rekacewicz, Philippe, 2000. *Guerillas and Paramilitary Forces in Colombia,* Le Monde Diplomatique. at http://mondediplo.com/maps

Rengert, George F., 1996. *The Geography of Illegal Drugs,* Boulder: Westview Press.

Reuter, Peter, 1996. "The Mismeasurement of Illegal Drug Markets," in *Exploring the Underground Economy,* W.E. Upjohn Institute for Employment Research, pp. 63–80.

Reuter, Peter, 1997. "Why Can't We Make Prohibition Work Better?," *Proceedings of the American Philosophical Society,* Vol. 141, No. 3.

Reuter, Peter, 1997. "Hawks Ascendant: The Punitive Trend of American Drug Policy," in McShane, Marilyn and Frank P. Williams III (eds.) *Drug Use and Drug Policy,* New York: Garland, pp. 365–402.

Reuter, Peter, 1998. "Foreign Demand for Latin American Drugs," in Joyce, Elizabeth and Carlos Malamud, (eds.) *Latin America and the Multinational Drug Trade,* Institute of Latin American Studies, pp. 23–43.

Rhodes, William, 1997. *What America's Users Spend on Illegal Drugs, 1988–1995.* Office of National Drug Control Policy.

Rice, John, 2000. "Dispute Rages Over Slain Cardinal," *Associated Press,* July 27.

Riley, Kevin Jack, 1996. *Snow Job? The War Against International Cocaine Trafficking,* New Brunswick: Transaction Publishers. (RAND).

Riley, Kevin Jack., 1997. "Crack, Powder Cocaine, and Heroin: Drug Purchase and Use Patterns in Six U.S. Cities." Washington, D.C.: National Institute of Justice.

Robinson, Linda, 1994. "Central America and Drug Trafficking," in Bagley, Bruce M., and William O. Walker III (eds.) *Drug Trafficking in the Americas,* New Brunswick: Transaction Publishers.

Robinson, L., 1998. "Is Colombia Lost to the Rebels?' *U.S. News and World Report,* 11 May, pp. 38–52.

Roche, Timothy, 2001. "Just another Day in a Bridge Town, *Time,* 11 June.

Rohter, Larry, 2000. "Weave of Drugs and Strife in Colombia," *New York Times,* April 21: A1.

Rosenberg, Matthew J. 2000. "Jamaica Struggles With Cocaine," *Associated Press,* February 10.

Sanabria, Harry, 1993. *The Coca Boom and Rural Social Change in Bolivia,* Ann Arbor: The University of Michigan Press.

Sassen, Saskia, 1994. "Place and Production in the World Economy," in *Cities in a World Economy,* London: Pine Forge, pp. 1–7.

Sauer, Carl Ortwin, 1963. *Land and Life: A Selection from the Writings of Carl Ortwin Sauer,* John Leighly (ed.), University of California Press.

Sayer, Andrew, 1982. "Explanation in Economic Geography: Abstraction versus Generalization, *Progress in Human Geography,* Vol. 6(1), pp. 68–88.

Sayer, Andrew, 1985. "The Difference that Space Makes," in D. Gregory and J. Urry (eds.) Social Relations and Spatial Structures, MacMillan, pp. 49–66.

Schemo, Diana Jean and Tim Golden, 1998. "Bogota Aid: To Fight Drugs or Rebels?" *The New York Times,* June 2: A1.

Schoenberger, Erica, 1992. "Self-Criticism and Self-Awareness in Research: A Reply to Linda McDowell, *Professional Geographer,* 44(2), pp. 215–218.

Schulz, Donald E. and Edward J. Williams. 1995. "Crisis or Transformation? The Struggle for the Soul of Mexico." in Schulz and Williams, eds. *Mexico Faces the 21st Century*. Westport, Connecticut: Greenwood Press.

Schusler, Ralph, 2000. "Drug Traffickers Threaten Stability," *Associated Press*, June 14.

Sequera, Vivian, 2000. "Colombia Militias Tax Drug Trade," *Associated Press*, January 10.

Shapiro, Bruce, 2000. "The Corruption of Col. James Hiett," *Salon.com news:* July 5.

Shepherd, William G., 1997. *The Economics of Industrial Organization*, Upper Saddle River, NJ: Prentice Hall.

Smith, Peter H., 1999. "Semiorganized International Crime: Drug Trafficking in Mexico," in *Transnational Crime in the Americas*, Farer, Tom (ed.), New York: Routledge. pp. 171–191.

Stafford, Howard A., 1972. "The Geography of Manufacturers," *Progress in Geography*, Vol. 4, pp. 181–215.

Stake, Robert E., 2000. "Case Studies," in Denzin and Lincoln (eds) *Handbook of Qualitative Research*. Thousand Oaks: Sage Publications.

Stevenson, Mark, 2000. "U.S. Czar: Drug War is no Real War," *Associated Press:* February 9.

Strauss, Anselm L., 1987. *Qualitative Analysis for Social Scientists*, Cambridge: Cambridge University Press.

Stutz, Frederick P., and Anthony R deSouza, 1998. *The World Economy*, Upper Saddle River: Prentice Hall.

Sullivan, Kevin and Mary Jordan, 2002. "Mexico Arrests Drug Boss," *Washington Post*, March 10: A1.

Swartz, Charles, 1996. "The Spatial Analysis of Crime," in Goldsmith, Victoe, Philip G. McGuire, John H. Mollenkopf, and Timothy A. Ross (eds.) *Analyzing Crime Patterns: Frontiers of Practice*, Thousand Oaks: Sage Publications.

Taaffe, Edward J., Howard L. Gauthier, and Morton E. O'Kelly, 1996. *Geography of Transportation*, Upper Saddle River: Prentice Hall.

Teichman, Judith, 1995. *Privatization and Political Change in Mexico*, Pittsburgh: University of Pittsburgh Press.

Texas Center for Border Economic and Enterprise Development, 2000. "Loaded Truck Crossings into Texas from Mexico, 1990–99," Laredo, TX: Texas A&M International University.

Thoumi, Francisco E., 1994. "The Size of the Illegal Drug Industry," in Bagley, Bruce M., and William O. Walker III (eds.) *Drug Trafficking in the Americas*, New Brunswick: Transaction Publishers.

Thoumi, Francisco E., 1995. *Political Economy & Illegal Drugs in Colombia*, Boulder: Lynne Rienner Publishers.

Thoumi, Fransisco E., 1999. "The Impact of the Illegal Drug Industry on Colombia" in *Transnational Crime in the Americas*, Farer, Tom (ed.), New York: Routledge. pp. 117–142.

Toro, Mar'a Celia, 1995. *Mexico's "War" on Drugs—Causes and Consequences*, Boulder: Lynne Rienner Publishers.

United Nations Drug Control Program, 2001. *Global Illicit Drug Trends*, www.undcp.org/global_illicit_drug_trends

United Nations Drug Control Program, 2001. "Colombia Country Profile," www.undcp.org/colombia.

U.S. Customs Service, 2000. "Windows of opportunity for Drug Smuggling," www.customs.gov/enforcmen/hardline.

U.S. Department of Commerce, 2002. *Colombia Country Commercial Guide,* U.S. Commercial Service.

U.S. Department of Justice, 1996. "The National Narcotics Intelligence Consumers Committee Report," www.usdoj.gov/dea/pubs/intel.

U.S. Department of Justice, 1996. "The South American Cocaine Trade," www.usdoj.gov/dea/pubs/intel/cocaine.

U.S. Department of Justice, 1996. "DEA Congressional Testimony," www.usdoj.gov /dea/pubs/cngrtest.

U.S. Department of Justice, 1998. "Patterns and Trends of Drug Use in Houston, Texas," www.tcada.tx.usa/research/currentrends/1998deahouston98.

U.S. Department of Justice, 1999–2000. "DEA Briefing Book," www.usdoj.gov/dea/briefingbook.

U.S. Department of Justice, 2000. "DEA Congressional Testimony," www.usdoj.gov/dea/pubs/cngrtest.

U.S. Department of Justice, 2000. "Federal Agents Dismantle International Drug Trafficking Organization," DEA Press Release, Dec. 14. www.usdoj.gov/dea/pubs/cngrtest.

U.S. Department of Justice, 2001. "Traffickers From Colombia," www.usdoj.gov/traffickers/colombia.

U.S. Department of Justice, 2001. "Traffickers From the Dominican Republic," www.usdoj.gov/traffickers/dr.

U.S. Department of Justice, 2001. "DEA Congressional Testimony," www.usdoj.gov/pubs/cngrtest.

U.S. Department of Justice, 2001. "Patterns and Trends of Drug Use in Houston, Texas," pp. 1–5. www.tcada.state.tx.us/research.

U.S. Department of Justice, 2002. "DEA News Release," June 27, www.usdoj.gov/pubs/cngrtest.

U.S. Department of State, 1997–2000. *International Narcotics Control Strategy Report,* Washington, DC: Government Printing Office.

U.S. International Trade Administration, 1991–1999. "U.S. Total Exports/Imports to/from Individual Countries." www.ita.doc.gov.

U.S. Sentencing Commission, 1995. "The Distribution and Marketing of Cocaine," in *Cocaine and Federal Sentencing Policy.* www.ussc.gov.

Valvanis, Stefan, 1968. "Lösch on Location," in R.H.T. Smith, E.J. Taaffe, and L.J. King (eds.), *Readings in Economic Geography: The Location of Economic Activity,* Chicago: Rand McNally, pp. 69–74.

Venkatesh, Sudhir, 2001. "The Financial Activity of a Modern American Street Gang," in Looking at Crime from the Street Level, U.S. Dept. of Justice.

Wai-chung Yeung, Henry, 1994. "Critical Reviews of Geographical Perspectives on Business Organizations and the Organization of Production: Towards a Network Approach," *Progress in Human Geography,* Vol. 18(4) pp. 460–490.

Wai-chung Yeung, Henry, 2000. "Organizing 'the Firm' in Industrial Geography I: Networks, Institutions and Regional Development," *Progress in Human Geography,* Vol. 24(2) pp. 301–15.

Walker, William O. III (ed.), 1996. "Introduction: Culture, Drugs, and Politics in the Americas," in *Drugs in the Western Hemisphere: An Odyssey of Cultures in Conflict*, Wilmington: SR Books. pp. xiii-xxvii.

Warren, K., 1970. *The British Iron and Steel Industry Since 1840*. London: Methuen.

Washington Post, 1996. "Cartels Fight Back in Mexico Drug War," May 26: 14A.

Watson, Cynthia A. 2000, "Civil-Military Relations in Colombia: a Workable Relationship or a Case for Fundamental Reform?" *Third World Quarterly*, Vol. 21, No. 3, pp. 529–548.

Weir, Carol, 1994. "Costa Rica and the Drug Trade," in Bagley, Bruce M., and William O. Walker III (eds.) *Drug Trafficking in the Americas*, New Brunswick: Transaction Publishers.

Westermeyer, Joseph, 1996. "Cultural Factors in the Control, Prevention, and Treatment of Illicit Drug Use," in Bickel, Warren K. and Richard J. DeGrandpre (eds.) *Drug Policy and Human Nature*, New York: Plenum Press.

Wheeler, James O., Peter O. Muller, Grant Ian Thrall, and Thomas J. Fik, 1998. *Economic Geography*, New York: John Wiley & Sons.

Williams, Phil, 2002. "Organizing Transnational Crime: Networks, Markets, and Hierarchies," in Williams, Phil and Dimitri Vlassis (eds). Combating Transnational Crime: Concepts, Activities and Responses. London: Frank Cass. Pp. 57–87.

Wilson, Scott, 2001. "Coca Invades Colombia's Coffee Fields," *Washington Post Foreign Service*, October 30: A17.

Zelinsky, Wilbur 1992. *The Cultural Geography of the United States*, Upper Saddle River: Prentice Hall.

Index

Z